stains noted 09/01/18

SO WE GO

SO WE GO

THE DAY MY FATHER DIED

MICHAEL HEMERY

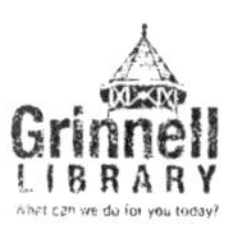

Deeds Publishing | Atlanta

Published by Deeds Publishing in Athens, GA
www.deedspublishing.com

Printed in The United States of America

Cover and text design by Mark Babcock

Library of Congress Cataloging-in-Publications data is available upon request.

ISBN 978-1-944193-81-2

Books are available in quantity for promotional or premium use. For information, email info@deedspublishing.com.

First Edition, 2016

10 9 8 7 6 5 4 3 2 1

Disclaimer

This is how the events were scribbled in my notebooks and my mind. I've done my best to tell it just as it happened, but if a hair or two is out of place, thanks for understanding. The names of only a few have been changed, but, for the most part, this is how we said goodbye.

To Mom and Stacie for being more powerful than any trial life can conjure. And to Kai and Vivienne for reminding me of the beauty in even the slightest breeze. You all make life something worth fighting for.

Our stories all end the same way; the difference is how we get there.

"He wants the BiPAP removed," Mom said. "Today."

It was 4:30 AM. I set the electric razor on the bathroom counter, forgetting to shut it off. My wife Stacie rushed into the bathroom, her eyes swollen with sleep. She clicked off the humming razor and touched my arm. Touched my fingers holding the phone.

"He's gone?" Stacie whispered.

I shook my head.

Our two-year-old son Kai fussed in the bedroom. "Momma," he said. "I want Momma." His voice was sweetness tinged with the light rasp of morning.

"We'll call off today, get subs to cover," I said. My throat was thick. "I'll have to run lesson plans to school, but we'll get Kai and come over as soon as I get back."

We owned the house directly behind my parents—a purchase ten years prior when we married. At the time we joked that my folks could do our laundry. Mow our lawn. Take care of us. My dad laughed his eyes closed the first Saturday morning Stacie and I stood in our pajamas, knocking on their back window because the smell of pancakes wafted through the backyards. We brought forks and grins. Mom shook her head after Pa unlocked the door. She said the move was a mistake as she pulled milk and flour out of the fridge to make more batter, cursing us the whole time.

Now the proximity allowed for hectic phone calls, sprints through the yard when there was a slip, a choke, an end.

Mom cried into the phone. "I don't know when," she said. "They might not let him. I mean, they don't just let people choose when they'll die. And I'm not ready."

I could hear her body shaking through the trembling of her voice.

"None of us are."

My dad spoke, garbled in the background. "I. Am." His voice was hollow, full of phlegm. His breathing machine, the BiPAP, began beeping a warning. His breathing was off. Three seconds. Four. The machine warned during the day, during meals, in the dead of sleep. It reminded us of its presence. Of the loss. Muscle. Breath. Of his emaciated core that lacked the strength to breathe in on its own. He kept speaking in one-second bursts. Clearer now. "They—have to." Beeping. "I can't keep—going." Beeping. Six. Seven more seconds. "I can't." The last words a gasp. A whisper. Near silent gags. He stopped speaking, so the machine returned to its rhythmic puffs. The beeping silenced. Air pushed in. Kept him alive.

1. All the Time in the World

Five hundred, maybe a thousand feet of bridge connected the hospital to the frozen custard stand. The morning after Stacie gave birth to Kai, my dad promised her a chocolate milkshake. He said she deserved it, that it'd go down smooth, much easier than the hospital's blanched broccoli and steamed carrot lunch. He extended his flattened hand away from his body like he was tracing the backside of a wave when he said "smooth," drawing out the vowels.

Despite the August heat I joined my dad for those five hundred, maybe a thousand feet. I needed to breathe in the humidity, stretch off the lack of sleep.

"God, he's perfect," Pa said. He turned his head when he spoke, walking a few paces ahead of me on the narrow cement walkway. Even though I was in my thirties, my dad still walked in front to shield me from a potential swerving car. He said at least I'd stand a chance.

I ran my hand along the low iron railing that protected pedestrians from the rocks of the shallow river below. "I can't get over those huge eyes," he said. "They just cut into you like he already understands everything."

My dad was the only one who hadn't held Kai. The nurses, my mom, and my cousin Kathleen, who drove from Virginia with her boyfriend Chris the moment she heard Stacie was in labor, had all cradled Kai in their arms. The nurses bounced him on their knees to ease his cries, and

Mom picked him up, nestling him into her shoulder after Stacie nursed him to sleep. Each time I offered Kai to my dad he shook his head. "Not yet. Later," he said. "We have all the time in the world."

As we walked across the bridge, I told him the experience seemed surreal—two fathers now walking across this bridge, not one. I mentioned that I was still nervous, being responsible for that tiny being that cried in the clear, plastic crib next to the hospital bed.

We walked swiftly, my legs moving too fast for comfort, a pace somewhere between jogging and walking. I spoke in breaths. Puffs between words. We moved quickly so we didn't neglect a cry, a murmur, a shift of the foot. Kai was less than one day old. Halfway across the bridge I thought I'd made a mistake by leaving him for ten minutes—that somewhere in those five hundred, maybe a thousand feet, I'd miss something.

When we arrived, the woman at the custard stand placed the perspiring plastic cup into a paper bag. She told me to be careful—to hold it from the bottom because on a day like today, it might soak through. We walked back to the hospital even quicker, the frozen custard melting in the brown bag. We didn't say much, but concentrated on our steps. The oncoming traffic was close, the air from the approaching trucks pulling our bodies toward the road, then pushing them back as they passed. My dad turned his head and said to be careful. That these people drive like assholes. That the little guy in that hospital room needed me.

Instead of watching the traffic, I concentrated on my dad's shoes. I lost myself in the repetition, the pattern, the simplicity of movement. Heel rocked to toe and over and over—the echo of motion propelling us. It would be so long before Kai could will his body to move this way, build the strength to cross the bridge the way we did. Father and son. I ran my hand along the rail again. Occasional bubbles of rust flaked away from my touch, floating to the river below like embers from a campfire. Heel toe. Heel toe. Heel toe. Heel toe. Slip.

My dad's back stuttered.

It was only a quiver, but the pattern gave way, barely enough to notice.

"What happened?" I asked.

He didn't answer immediately, but breathed—his shoulders rising and falling. He didn't stop. We were halfway across the bridge. I looked away from his shoes at the river beneath us. It'd been particularly dry so only trickles of water meandered between rocks and fallen tree trunks.

I asked again.

He shouted over the clamor of traffic that it was his back. "The damn thing has just been fucked up lately." He straightened as he walked.

"Did you lift something?"

He shook his head.

A large heron flew from a nearby tree limb to the river below, poking his beak between the rocks. With so little water the fish were easy targets. The bird tilted his head back and flapped his massive wings. He repeated the action several more times before flying away, following the river's curve.

The perspiration from the milkshake disintegrated most of the bag. I asked my dad if he wanted to stop, take a break. He said, "Stacie needs that milkshake before it's soup."

"She can wait; it'll be fine," I said.

My dad was beyond fit—his body toned and muscular from years of physical labor. He was also beyond handsome—his salt-and-pepper hair only complemented his striking dark face, soft eyes and smile that spread naturally across his face. Whenever Mom's friends would mention him or he'd come through the room from working outside, they'd blush when he said hello. And if he ever graced a room by speaking French, his native language, he could melt any woman.

But on the bridge something in his perfect body had failed him. I asked if he was going to be okay, if he needed to see a doctor, how long it had been this way. He continued walking. I chased after him, ringing off questions. We still walked at the same breakneck pace. He shouted back to me. Said it'd been "fucked up" for a few months, that he'd see a doctor if it didn't get better, not to be concerned. "Just worry about that little guy upstairs," he shouted back to me. "He's the best."

I watched his every step, no longer as a distraction, but in case his body shape shifted again, twisting from the narrow walk into the street. I clutched the milkshake bag in my left hand so my right was free to catch my father and protect him from the traffic. Heel toe. Cars. Heel toe. Cars. Heel toe. Heel toe heel toe heel toe heel toe. Five hundred, maybe a thousand.

When we reached the hospital he let me find an open door, most locked for security. He waited on the sidewalk so he didn't have to walk as far, adding more strain to his back. I waved him over after I found an entry.

When I handed Stacie the milkshake she thanked my dad, asking if he wanted to hold Kai now.

"Not quite yet," he said, breathing hard as he lowered himself into the chair. My mom said to quit being stupid. She slapped him on the back of the head and said he wasn't going to break him. My dad flinched, flattening his hair. Mom lifted Kai out of the crib, told Pops to make a cradle, and placed my boy in my dad's arms.

That memory of the hospital room is clearer than anything I know to be true. The one wall was all windows, the light sharper than any late autumn sun that perfectly silhouettes brightly-colored leaves. It didn't smell like hospital, but baby—sweet, new. Stacie sucked on the straw of her milkshake, cheeks pulled in. The warmth of slurps and baby coos. There was music, a mix of "newborn" songs I'd prepared for the recovery room. Laughter. And tears. The moment Kai was placed in his arms, my dad began to cry. Mom laughed, said he was being silly. "Perfect," he said. Repeated. "Perfect." Kai stared at my dad while he cried. Unblinking. He held my son until the nurse came to run a test. Until the tears dried on his cheeks and the sun changed into something else.

2. Telephone

How she said the letters like one word. *Alias*. As if this wasn't happening to him, but someone else. Someone more deserving. Eric Blair died of tuberculosis, not George Orwell. It's so much easier to kill a stranger.

How I asked her to repeat it.

How I told her to hang on. Turned up the phone's volume.

How that must have felt, my dad driving them both home from the clinic, having to hear it again. But slower. Each letter a puff of air from the top of the throat.

How ALS sounds when divided up, each letter given attention.

How the doctor told them. He wasn't positive. But preliminary tests. He briefly searched on the Web. It seemed to be. He recommended a neurologist. Didn't say much more.

How I could hear Mom tighten in the pauses.

How I asked for more, almost casually, almost like he had a cold, an eye spasm, a torn ligament that could be repaired with a surgery, a tweak, a cut and a tie. Almost like he'd be okay.

How I made her say it again.

How she said, "Goddammit, Mike," before whispering, "Lou Gehrig's."

How she didn't say *disease*. Like she didn't want anyone to hear. Like if the tongue didn't click the roof of the mouth, snake through the teeth, open, then return, his limbs would begin to function properly. His back would straighten. Like without the word, the disease itself couldn't manifest into anything proper. Anything at all.

How the first thought I had was a joke from Denis Leary, a comedian I heard in a friend's car during high school. "Poor Lou Gehrig. Died of Lou Gehrig's disease.

How the hell did he not see that coming?"

How I laughed when I heard the punch line. My friend put four dollars of gas into his car, lit cigarette in his mouth, and left the engine running while he pumped. I told him to shut it off or he'd blow us all to kingdom come. He said just listen to the CD. He said a little danger reminds us we're alive.

How I laughed again, no longer listening to the CD, because I was terrified a spark from a quick drag might dance into the gas line, light us up.

How now I sat in my car, two blocks from that gas station. Ten years later. Parked between two windowless full-sized vans. One red. One white.

How I wanted to yawn, stretch those vans away.

How I shut off the engine because Mom told me that carbon monoxide seeps into the car when not moving.

How you can kill yourself when you're not even trying.

How two minutes prior Stacie repeated our takeout order before she slid out of the car. Just to be sure she had it right.

How I told her to hang on, because I had a gift card in my wallet. I'd forgotten it was there and worried it would expire soon. I said the word *worried.*

How $15 mattered.

How Kai was silent in the back seat. We drove to quiet him. Figured the movement would lull him to sleep.

How all we needed was a momentary break. A few minutes. Respite from the crying.

How.

How my mother was still there, hushed, except for the air being pinched by her nose. My phone amplifying the intakes of breath. The tears that stream the cheeks get all the attention, but never the ones that prevent us from breathing; you can't wipe those away.

How when I pushed her further, asked about next steps, fixes, answers, she breathed heavier.

How air is worse than words.

How I continued to press.

How she answered.

How I repeated the answers.

How the words *fatal, incurable* sounded when I said them aloud. Like the anchor on the local evening news who appears once a week for the *Health Report.* Swirling blue graphics behind blond hair. She's somewhat overweight for an anchor. Ironic, I'd always thought, that she was the health reporter. Maybe she's just not what we expect. When she speaks, she's abrasive. When she mentions children with cancer or twenty-somethings with HIV, her words aren't whispered or quiet. There is no rise in her voice at the end of sentences. No hope. She says the word *disease* like she means it.

How I've cried during the *Health Report.* Said words like, *So sad, Not right.*

How sports or weather is always on right after.

How easy it is to forget when it's someone else.

How repeated words lingered in a car with a silenced child and a van on either side and no noise, not even the white noise of traffic because the windows were rolled up, and a phone so loud—the volume bars all the way to the right—and there were no clever segues or puns or baseball scores, and goddamn if only it would have been raining or snowing or windy so there could have been something, anything else to drag down the words *fatal* and *incurable* like pollen, goldenrod, wisps of irritants that can't be caught in the hand because they're too soft, slippery, finding escape in slits of tightly pressed fingers, only muted when something wet and heavier than them, the first pellets of a spring storm, a deluge from a pall of dark clouds, catch them off guard, adding weight, battering them to the ground where they can't hurt anyone anymore.

How I could hear my father in the background of the conversation.

How he asked something from the driver's seat.

How far away his voice seemed.

How quickly distance can grow in a relatively small moment.

How I think he asked if Kai was doing okay.

How we sat in silence for several more seconds, my phone pressed closely to my ear.

How he then asked something about dying, maybe forgetting Mom was still on the phone.

How my mother didn't repeat his question, relay it back to me like *telephone,* that game in elementary school where one kid says something to the next and you wait to see how the message transforms itself because of mishearings. The first time I played in Mrs. Hudako's class, I misunderstood the directions. I thought we were *supposed* to change the words. To intentionally disturb the order of language. Change what was said into something more interesting. Something better. So when Kate whispered into my ear, "Potato pie is fun to eat," I paused. Thought for a second. Leaned into Jenny, cupping my hand around my mouth and her ear, a protective tunnel so no one else would know.

How I said, "Apple pie is made of meat."

How Jenny looked at me, cocked her eyebrow, and continued to spread the message. At least ten more kids. Ten more changes. I waited to see what would be said. But when Mark stood up at the end of the line and said, "Apple pie is made of meat," I didn't understand.

How easily it was to pinpoint the weak link. Jenny pointing. Kate pointing.

How I pleaded my case, questioning the validity of a game that prided itself on redundancy and accuracy, discarding the importance of deliberate change.

How I thought that's what we were supposed to do.

How the teacher shook her head.

How we had to start again, play the right way this time.

How she looked at me when she said the word *right*.

How Mrs. Hudako whispered into Jon's ear.

How Kate whispered, "Snow can quiet a mountain."

How I cupped my hand around Jenny's ear.

How this happened at least ten more times.

How Mark stood.

How clearly he said the words.

Like they meant anything at all.

3. Sure

While my father waited for the test results from the neurologist, his back gave way more rapidly; it went from a pause to a limp to a hand on a thigh, like a buttress, architecture for the ache. He and Mom stopped walking the neighborhood past our house, down the street, through the elementary school parking lot and around again. In the winter Stacie and I would hear a battery of sound against our front windows, then giggles from the sidewalk. When we'd pull open the blinds, fresh snowballs slid down the glass, my parents running down the street, loose snow kicking up in their wake. It never grew old.

Now they didn't call for our dog to join them; she sniffed underneath the closed closet door where her leash hung, then turned back to the living room, circled, and resigned herself to the floor with a huff. There were no more pit stops for a beer or quips that I really should touch up the paint on my garage door. "What kind of shanty you running here?" Pa would ask. I'd tell him not to worry about it—that no one but him even noticed. Without his scrutiny it peeled unchecked by anyone.

The doctor said it would be a few days, maybe weeks to know for sure. Though, he corrected, with ALS there is no *for sure*. The only way to diagnosis the disease with any certainty is through autopsy. So the doctor pricked my dad's fingers and toes with electricity, testing the nerves to see if they answered back in electric echoes. The nurses joked with my dad during the exam, saying something about the cold water he submerged his feet in for more accurate testing results. He laughed back. The doctor wrote down some numbers on a clipboard and said he'd call with results. To just wait.

But he couldn't just wait. It wasn't in his fiber. Instead, my father pumped air into the tires of his bike. It'd been years since he'd ridden competitively—sixty-mile treks to Lake Erie from our suburban Cleveland home. When he purchased his first racing bike, he trained every night, riding the oval of our neighborhood—lap after lap after work, pushing speed and distance, ignoring the stop signs. He bought an odometer and speedometer to keep track. To know for sure.

The neighbors soon noticed my dad's circuit. Every summer evening dozens of boys and their fathers emerged from garages on bikes—mountain bikes, ten speeds, even tricycles—as soon as my dad began circling. They all wanted a piece of the action. Of my dad's speed. On any given night dozens of bikes trailed behind him, a *peloton*, a platoon of riders, jockeying for position to outrun my father. I rode in this pack on my red BMX with the nubby tires, listening to the older kids promise they'd overtake him. Tonight. One by one they'd stand on their bikes, pumping their pedals like pistons, trying to pass him. My dad never had to stand, but wore yellow Oakley goggles and a helmet, riding with his head down to minimize resistance. His legs moved in a patient rhythm, never frantic nor desperate.

No one ever caught him—never even came close. He was too fast. Too smart. Saved his energy for the uphill. Harnessed gravity on the slope. I loved that my dad could outride anyone in the neighborhood; I never wanted another boy's father to pass him, never wanted him to slow down. He rode for himself, but he was aware of the steady hunt in his periphery, waiting for him to slip.

We'd ride for hours, until the boys and their fathers were called home for dinner, dissolving into garages and warmly-lit kitchens. I'd tired long before, sitting at my usual spot by the stop sign, bike on its side, pulling out blades of grass, cheering on my father as he shot by, head down, smiling.

My father rode solitarily until sunset. He'd decelerate for his final pass, waving for me to join him, so I'd rush to right my bike, pushing hard on the pedals to keep up. Pa always rode upright for the final run, gloves unsnapped, hands not on the handlebars. One hand gripped a water bottle, while the other reached across the road to support my back, pushing me along as we rode in tandem like a catamaran. He'd chuckle as I struggled to maintain his now slower pace, and say, "Faster, faster," as we took our victory lap back home. "Exhaustion is mental," my dad would say. "Whenever you're tired, you can still give more." So I pushed myself to be near him, to ride in stride with my father. Every night when we'd arrive home, he'd unclip his shoes from the pedals and hold my hand in the air, shouting "Victory, victory," loud enough for the neighbors to hear.

At age sixty, as we awaited the results of a test that would suggest the onset of a paralyzing disease that would ultimately cripple my father, confining him to one chair in his living room, a disease that had already prevented him from walking more than a few steps without exhaustion, a disease that was more cruel than anything I'd ever known, my father discovered he was still able to ride his bike with ease.

So he rode.

Each night he took to his former circuit, but now expanded its course to his old walking route. He rode past our house, up the street, through the elementary school parking lot, and around again—every night after work, until a familiar sunset called him home. He wore the same helmet and glasses he'd donned years ago, but now slightly faded and washed out. When I mowed my front yard I'd linger by the street, waiting for him to come by. He was still so fast. I'm sure the muscle loss compound-

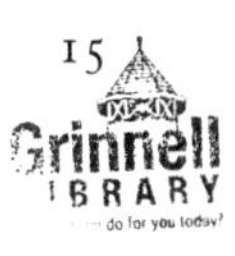

ed with years of not riding slightly impeded his speed, but as I maneuvered my mower up and down the curve of the ditch, hacking away at crabgrass and clover, he sped by in the same blur of color I remembered as a child, nodding his head, smiling.

He rode his bike everywhere—the park, convenience store, Grandma's house. He was fine as long as he didn't stop. When his feet rested on the cement, his back caved again, forcing him to use the bike's long bar for support. One afternoon as I drove to the grocery store to pick up cheddar cheese I'd forgotten to purchase the day before, I passed my father on one of our city's busy roads. He rode on the sidewalk. He never rode on the sidewalk. He always said it was too slow, full of garbage that could pop the skinny tires of his racing bike, so we always pedaled the streets. Men in cars would honk and curse at us, trying to pass. He said we had every right to be there. Once, when my dad was in his twenties, a man in a truck gave him shit for being on the road as he biked to work. The man swerved at him, clipped his handlebar, then accelerated with his middle finger out the window. My dad pedaled hard to catch up at a traffic light where he told the man to "fuck off" before kicking in the passenger door with his steel-toed boots. He took off down side streets to work. Smiling, I'm sure.

I honked my horn as I slowed my car, waving down my dad. He didn't look up. I honked again. He raised his head. There were so many tears, his face slick.

I turned down the first side road, leaving my car in the street. My dad had already caught up and straddled the bar, using the handlebars for support. I met him on the sidewalk. His face was streaked red. When I hugged him, his breath hinted red wine. We held one another, motionless, except for the slight tremors from his back and heaves from his chest.

The street was lined with suburban houses, twenty feet from the sidewalk, and as we remained locked, I wondered if anyone watched. If anyone peered from their windows as I hugged him on his bike in the middle of the afternoon in front of their homes.

My dad pulled away from me, swung his leg over the bike, and used the bar as a perch.

"How did you know to look for me?" he asked.

I explained the coincidence, groceries, how it wasn't intended.

He still cried, using the back of his hand to wipe his nose.

"Maybe it's not ALS," I said. "We have to wait for the tests. The Internet said the back is usually the last thing to go, so maybe this is something else. Something that can be fixed. None of the other symptoms match—no shaky hands or tripping or anything." Failure of the outer extremities is one of the first symptoms. The core is the last to go, except for a rare few.

He breathed hard, adjusting himself on the bar. "Don't tell your mom," he said. He raised his hand. It quivered. "But my right hand shakes. A lot. It started a few months ago, but it shakes. It's harder to pick up small shit at work. It took me a fucking half hour to deal with some small screws in the computer the other day. Should have taken two minutes. Goddamn half hour." My dad was in charge of the computer systems for the local school district. He worked his way up from being a janitor to being in charge of all the district's computers. He lowered his hand. "Don't tell your mother. She doesn't need this."

His tears slowed. His breathing followed.

"But maybe that's all just something else, Pa. We can't lose hope until we know for sure. I read something about Lyme's disease having similar symptoms."

There was some silence. His neurons were failing as we spoke.

A car drove by.

"I'm not scared of dying," he said. He wiped his face. "I'm not. I had a good life. Worked hard. Goddamn, I worked hard." My father worked since he was thirteen, beginning as a pressman for little pay and too much work. His job as a janitor overlapped with the printing, but he had to get out because the stress of the job was killing him. So after working all day on the presses, he'd clock in for night shifts at the school. He'd worry about each job, making himself sick at night: Did he lock down the rolls of paper, clean the school thoroughly enough? "And what do I have to show for it? What?" He could retire in four months. He'd never taken off more than two weeks in a row his entire life. He accumulated hundreds of sick days. He never stopped.

He eventually accepted the full-time evening janitor job at a local elementary school when I was thirteen. I asked my mom if we could visit one night. I then understood what it meant to work like my dad. He kissed me on the head when I arrived, but for the remainder of the visit I literally broke a sweat sprinting from room to room to keep up. He spoke quickly, moving a vacuum over carpeting, scrubbing desks, and wiping chalkboards. I asked if he could slow down to talk for a few minutes. He said in order to get everything done, he couldn't stop. He always skipped dinner. He had to keep moving.

"But we're not there, and you've had a good life. And are going to keep having a good life."

"It's not death I'm upset about. I had the best life with you and your mom and now Stacie and Kai. It's not death. I worry about your mother and how she'll get by without my paycheck. The house is so much work. She doesn't need that. She doesn't deserve that."

I could feel my own tears welling, but I swallowed them. I cry so easily, but I had to be someone else. I had to be him.

"Pa, we can't even talk about that right now. That is so far away. This can't be it."

"I ask God why. I mean, when your mom miscarried before having you, I was so angry with God. I hated Him. And then you were born. So there was a reason. There is always a reason. I just can't figure this one out. I don't understand.

"And I regret a lot. A lot of what I'm not. I should have went to college and made more money so it would have been easier. There is so much regret."

I could smell the wine on his breath more clearly now. He closed his eyes. Held them shut, pressing fingers into his sockets.

"Pa, there is *nothing* to regret. You gave me a better life than anyone could wish for. We had so much happiness together. I can't imagine anything better."

"I worked too much."

"You did what you had to for us."

He began to cry again. He never cried.

"It's okay. I'll be okay," he said between sobs. "This is just what happens when you get old. You think about all the things you could have done differently. I wish I had more for your mother."

"More than love?"

He shook his head and whispered, "No." He whispered it again. He took a deep breath, his shoulders rising and falling, the bike wobbling as he shifted his weight. "No. This just wasn't the plan. This wasn't how it was supposed to be."

"We still don't know."

My dad looked up from the ground, then closed his eyes. Opened them. "I do."

I looked into the window of the house directly behind him, trying to latch my eyes on the distance—on something that would prevent tears, which would only make it harder on him.

"That's why I haven't held Kai much. I'm scared. I don't want my hands or my arms to give. To drop him. It's not because I don't love him."

There were lace curtains on the second floor of the home. White. They made two swaying arcs and shifted when the late-summer wind pushed through the open window. I could see wallpaper—white with some sort of pattern, polka dots or maybe tiny baskets or watering cans. I moved my eyes to the small front porch with red rails that matched the shutters. Then to my dad's face. Dry now. Still staring at me.

"I'm okay," he said. He promised.

"It's a lot to try and wrap our heads around."

"But it'll be okay. Whatever happens. It'll be okay."

We remained on that sidewalk for another half hour talking about symptoms, wrong diagnoses, Mom, and Kai's hatred of "tummy time." He mentioned work that needed to be done to the house and how Stacie and I would take care of Mom. I paused too long before adding, "And you."

The September wind grew colder. I shivered, and he said I should get inside so *I* didn't catch cold. He said Mom would be worried why he was gone so long. He'd told her he was riding his bike to the video store. I assured him that I'd call her to let her know that he was okay.

I hugged him again, rubbed his back, still strong. Before the decay began stripping off years of muscle, shoulder blades striking through skin. Before he became emaciated. Before. At that moment I hugged the sturdy back of a man that worked tirelessly for forty-some years to provide for his family. A back that dug out his entire home's foundation with a shovel. Lifted, carried, hauled. There's a photo of the two of us removing a bush from the front of my home when we first moved in. In the image I'm tired and filthy. He's holding a shovel and smiling. He loved his body when he pushed it beyond exhaustion.

We pulled apart.

He told me he loved me.

I told him I loved him.

I offered to load his bike in the back of my car to drive him home. He shook his head, braced himself on the handlebars and swung his leg over his bike. "I need to ride." He put one foot on the pedal. "While I still can."

The wind rustled the curtain.

He told me again not to mention any of this to Mom and that he loved me. He heaved his body forward, fighting for balance on the slight incline, and pedaled. He didn't smile, riding not for pleasure anymore, but necessity. I returned to my car to watch his bike glide over the sidewalk, nearing the peak of the hill. On the bike he moved with the same fluidity as before. No trace of neurological rot or struggle. He rode with the determination that left the neighborhood trailing behind him many years before. After he crested and disappeared at the top of the hill, I continued to sit in my car, checking the horizon for movement, until I was sure he was gone.

4. Results

Positive.

"All by yourself today?" I inquired as the man behind the counter placed my bagels into a paper bag. I didn't want to be pleasant, but kindness was a gag reflex. The lights in the bagel shop seemed dim, like the store wasn't supposed to be open yet, like I was somewhere I wasn't supposed to be. A scant selection of only plain and blueberry bagels sat in the wire bins behind the counter.

The man with an overgrown goatee chuckled. He put two more bagels into the bag, then laughed again, too loudly for the nearly-empty room. A man in a mesh baseball hat sitting near the window looked up from his coffee. He cleared something from his front teeth, then returned to the newspaper that sprawled on the table.

"No, the other two are in the back supposedly finishing up the bagels," he said. He craned his neck to look into the back room. "But Lord knows they don't make any attempt to hurry, that's for darn sure."

He was always this way—perky.

"Coffee this morning?" he sang, dragging out the "ng."

I wanted to tell him. The whole thing. The two and a half years of the disease—one of which was complete and utter misery. The hell Pa and Mom experienced every fucking day. I wanted to tell him I was picking up breakfast because I figured despite the events that were unfolding, we'd need some sort of sustenance if we were going to make it. That my dad was preparing to have his BiPAP breathing machine removed. That I was about to lose my dad. I wanted to tell him what it felt like to know that the man you loved more than any other man in the world was going to be dead before the day ended. I wanted to look at him from darkened eyes that cried the entire drive to school, in my classroom as I put copies of worksheets out for my students and wrote a note for the substitute teacher that ended in *Thank You*, and on the drive back. I wanted to tell him that the recipient of this breakfast was death.

I smiled. "No, I'm all set."

Reflexes.

"You have yourself a good day," he said, looking at the name on my credit card before handing it back, "Michael."

Michael Daniel Hemery. My dad's name carved between mine.

I slipped the plastic into my wallet. Grabbed the bag. Nodded and said, "You too."

5. Believe It

Mom's suggestion came after we told the family—the news passed on. After the sobs—the ones that uncontrollably shake the body into convulsions like actors in movies on the edges of beds. My bed. I'd always chalked those films up to overacting and exaggeration. But I was mistaken—never before had I reason to double over with chest a rivet gun, hammering out tears. Semiautomatic moments—the thought of a funeral squeezing the trigger until the eyes dry heaved with nothing left to offer. Stacie happening upon me. Rubbing my back. Her eyes red. Saying she didn't know what to say. So we said nothing. Sometimes touch was enough.

It came after I walked the sidewalks of my neighborhood over and over with headphones crushing my ears, the lyrics to Against Me's "Up the Cuts" somehow forever coupled with the news. "Are you restless like me?" I listened on repeat for no good reason except maybe hoping the repetition would drown out reality for a bit.

After we had time to sit, stare through the nothingness of a wall; a chair; Kai in his crib swatting at the mobile my parents just bought him, colorful clowns dangling upside down, holding on by the curve of a slipper, spinning to a melancholy tune, not quite sad, but more a thoughtful, rainy afternoon; the dog nudging her empty food bowl, the metal clanging against the tile. It may have rained, thundered, lit the sky up with lightning looking for the quickest path to extinguish itself. But no one cared to notice. We all lingered in not-quite-numbness, but in exhaustion. I excused myself when Mom invited us to dinner that Sunday, right after. I lost it in their bathroom, trying to wash my face before returning to hotdogs and potato salad, and to prevent my lip from quivering from anything true.

Sometime after those moments, Mom pulled apple cobbler from the oven and said, "Just because they say it's ALS doesn't mean we have to believe it."

I paused for a moment, then asked, "What does that even *mean*?" My dad focused on his hand's grip of the fork.

"We don't have to believe them. It could be something else."

"But the doctors said—" I began.

"Even if it is. We don't have to live that way." She shook her head, setting the steaming glass dish on the trivet sitting on the table. "It's hot," she said. "Be careful."

Kai slept through much of the meal in his car seat at our feet. He began to whimper before he fully awoke, his eyelids tightening shut. Pops said we should place him on a chair next to the table so he'd feel included, even if he was still sleeping. "He's part of this now," Pa said. So we moved Kai to the table and tried to follow Mom's advice. We evaded, skirted, discussed breast feeding and baby toys instead of diagnoses. After dinner Pa stood, using the table as leverage as he pushed himself up from the bench that circled half the table. He worked his way to the sink, plate in one hand, the other hand borrowing support from the chair, refrigerator, then cabinet handle. He rested against the counter. Mom said to leave the dishes. She'd deal with them after we left. Since I could remember, Pa always washed dishes promptly after dinner—one of my earliest photos is me clinging to his pant leg while he scrubbed dishes clean. On Thanksgiving, while Grandpa talked about snow blowers and I waited my turn for my cousin's Gameboy, Pa would disappear for an hour, dishes clanking in the kitchen. He told me repeatedly growing up, "Since your mother works all day and then has to cook, it's the least I can do." He also vacuumed up dog hair every evening and tended to the laundry. "There's no such thing as 'man's work,'" he'd tell me. "You each do your part to make it work."

Now at the kitchen counter my dad cleared his throat. "I think your mom's right. We don't have to believe it. We don't have to live that way." He suggested we move to the living room. Hand on counter. Chair. Wall.

"Is it denial?" Stacie asked as we walked through the backyard on the way home, me swinging the empty car seat and Stacie cradling Kai in her arms. "Because they're both always so grounded. They know the right thing to do, usually. But they need to make plans to outfit the house for him and figure out his job. He can't keep working. They can't just pretend this isn't happening."

I knew she was right, but I trusted my folks—and they never were much for convention. All the kids in my elementary school used standard-issue Texas Instrument calculators, but my dad bought me an HP. There was no equal sign, and the keys weren't spongy like other calculators, but clicked when I pressed them, allowing me to work more quickly than my friends. My entire life my folks did everything slightly off, just a bit and enough to notice. And they did everything together: vacations, dinners, and even grocery shopping—my dad would wander to the cleaning supplies, then magazines, while Mom foraged for produce and meat. But they were there together. Because they said it was better. Because it was.

No, this was something more than denial. There was no pretending—I knew they'd still drive downtown together for doctors' appointments and heed the advice of the therapist and contact the ALS Association when they required consult. They'd received notice. They understood the memo from corporate. But this was a choice on how to live every day in the confines of their world as his body's neurons clicked off like the lights in an office building slated for demolition.

Mom and Pa decided to bustle about this now darkened, abandoned building together the next day and the next, rifling through old files in the quiet of the space, tossing wads of paper at each other, running into the corners of desks and giggling at their bruises. They'd carry on that way, admiring the view from their windows and holding one another for warmth until the first bolts of dynamite ignited the ground floor, sending the two of them collapsing into the dust and ashes of laughter, together.

6. Rather

Most of my family, all of my wife's family, the man in our neighborhood who we only see on Halloween as he pulls his princess daughter around in a plastic wagon, the rest of the adult neighbors, the whole cast of *Cheers*, the woman who checks people in at the rec center, my old minister, the whole congregation (except for the kids), the ninety-something-year-old friend of the family who performs an extreme stunt like skydiving or motorcycle racing each year for his birthday, my ex-girlfriends, their families, everyone I've friended on Facebook, those I haven't, the class of 1995, 1999, anyone I ever had a crush on who ignored my advances, the girl who broke up with me by not returning my calls and disappearing like she'd been abducted, the older couple in the car in front of me at the ATM machine because they laugh so hard I can hear them several feet away because they look so happy when they say something about needing to get that case of beer and not even because, sports heroes, music stars, my friends' parents, anyone in the circus, my former bosses, my current ones, the dark-haired woman who works at Target who flirts with me saying she'll invite me to dinner someday even though I'm married and even though she has kids my age, my coworker who emailed and asked about my dad and then emailed again when I didn't respond pointing out I avoided the question, her ex-husband, her current husband, her father, her mother, my dad's friends who said they couldn't come over because it was too hard to see him that way, every member of the FDA, the Middle East, Africa, Asia, Russia, Sarah Palin, John Kasich, Dane Cook, Angelina Jolie, Madonna, the NFL, my fifth-grade teacher with her long brown hair and stories about God, my best friends, their parents, their brothers, the guy who sold me my new video camera because he didn't know I'd be using it to tape my dad's last movements and interactions or why I insisted on asking over and over if the video would look okay in low light because I knew eventually that's how the lights would be surrounding my dad and not even because, the mailman, the garbage men, the twins who worked at the local bagel shop who were training to be dancers and would undercharge us every Saturday because we were regulars, their parents, the staff of Best Buy, the woman who tried to charge me more than she should have for my wife's new sewing machine, the mechanic who tried to tell me I needed thousands of dollars of work on my car until my dad showed up and asked to see the problem specifically and the man fumbled and stuttered and said it must have been a mistake, the Sears employee who sold my dad a metal cabinet for his garage with a huge dent in the side two months after he was diagnosed (he didn't return it because he said it still worked and it didn't matter because he didn't need everything to be perfect), everyone in the fishing village in Fécamp, France, where my dad grew up, the waiter who practiced his English on us when we returned to visit, hunters, fishermen, politicians, insurance agents, lawyers because, the doctor who told my dad it was ALS, the specialist who spoke to him like he was seven in a high-pitched happy voice commenting on his new cane that opened into a chair so he could sit when his legs grew weak after a few steps, the doctor who delivered Kai, the nurse who stayed with us during the entire nineteen-hour labor cheering Stacie on and then lingering in the room after we left because they were shorthanded and she had to mop and sterilize the room, my mom's friend who swears she has seen the ghost of her son after he shot himself in his car, grandmothers—all of them, grandfathers too, Maria the elderly French woman at the Saturday farmer's market who is said to have healing powers is said never to have eaten in a restaurant because she speaks so quietly because she sat with my parents and me for forty-five minutes and asked my father about France because they spoke French together and he had to lean forward to hear her quiet voice because she supposedly healed a woman at the market by praying for her because she freezes so much produce she can sustain herself during the winter months because she parked in the handicapped spot next to my dad—each with their handicapped tags hanging from the rearview mirrors, not even because, the living authors of my favorite books, everyone else at the Fourth of July picnic, the man who has worked at the hardware store since I was a kid—the one my dad and I stole a drip valve from because they didn't sell them individually and we would have had to buy the whole unit so we looked at one another and nodded and I slipped the tiny piece of metal into my pocket, the optometrist because he made a pass at Stacie while he told her to blink blink not even because, librarians, CEOs, laborers, teachers, gas station attendants, business people, bankers, George W. Bush because he rallied against life-saving (my dad-saving) stem cell research you motherfucking goddamn worthless piece of shit because because because because, clerks, factory workers, pilots, barbers, owners, sellers, buyers, my great aunt who rested her hands on my dad's shoulders when she hugged him on Father's Day causing him to nearly collapse, my grandma, grandpa (both of them), aunt, uncle, cousins, extended cousins, you. Sitting there now with moisture in your mouth, tongue able to move to the roof of your mouth. Breathe. Do it again. Move your arm. Legs. Maybe don't even move them, but know that you can. Breathe again. Feel what breath feels like. I'd rather it was you that had his disease. Not even because.

7. Click, Buzz

My whole life, my dad trained me not to say goodbye. Before the diagnosis, he always ended a phone call with, "Click, buzz." When I'd say *goodbye*, he'd correct me. Saying *goodbye* is permanent. Forever. *Click* was the sound of the phone hanging up; *buzz* is what you're left with when the other person's connection stops. "And that's what it is," he said. "Simple mechanics. Click. Buzz. We're still there. We'll see each other again. Talk again. So say what it really is. And it's not goodbye."

After the positive identification of the disease we began our dance on the phone, trying to discern what to say after a call. Despite years of corrections, I'd still sometimes slip. G*oodbye.* I was now careful how I ended things—fearful he wouldn't correct, let the terminal remain. Because that's what it really was.

He never called much before—I don't think he ever understood the need for small talk or chatting. Say what you had to say. And since we lived so close, he preferred to walk through the yard to show me his new iPod or discuss the leak from my gutters. But now he called so much more. He asked about the dog, if she was stir crazy because of the winter months. He called Kai a "little sucker" for not gaining enough weight, for being a lazy eater, distracted by sounds, the dog, a creak in the house. "Don't make me come over there," he said. "I'll let that little sucker have it for not eating." Then he laughed. Pa had a cold so his airways remained clogged with thick mucus. When he coughed the previous night on the phone, it sounded muffled. I thought he covered the receiver, but Mom said it was his stomach. The muscles were deteriorating, disappearing, forcing the coughs into slight releases.

"The *San Francisco Chronicle* is in a shithouse of trouble," he told me on another call. I listened for one of the first times to my dad. It used to be the other way. I'd go for hours, talking about school, music, video games. He'd listen, never interjecting much. But now he had so much to say. Maybe just in case.

He said he understood why newspapers were failing. "They're expensive and messy. When I used to work at Gowe Printing there were the solvents and ink and other garbage in that paper. It's all just such a waste." I interjected a few "un-huhs," but remained mostly silent because I wanted him to talk. I wanted him to say what he needed to. He laughed for a bit, a surface laugh—something like a warm up. "And who the fuck needs all those ads?" My dad had recently cancelled his *Cleveland Plain Dealer* subscription, except for Sundays, which he kept for my mom. "The paper is now just ads. Fucking Value City bullshit. I don't want a thirty-five dollar couch. No one should have a thirty-five dollar goddamn couch." He told me he missed his old couch, the soft leather one with the matching love seat. "I could sleep on that couch. Not like this new one all stiff and cloth. That old couch, now that was a nice couch. Smooth. This one is all rough and scratchy. And it wasn't cheap. I can only imagine what $35 feels like, all plywood and foam." I heard him smacking the pillow.

I asked why he'd sleep on the couch. He told me that wasn't the point. It was the fact that he *could* if he needed to. Then he said, "Ah well, who gives a shit anyhow? Fuck the newspapers, right?" He laughed from the belly like he was really pleased with himself. Although there was a strain in this laugh, it was solid—not muffled like the coughs, but more genuine. It reached various degrees of pitch, then wheezed before rolling into something deeper. He repeated it: "Fuck 'em, right?" Right, I said. I let him laugh.

"And the goddamn skunks. I swear last year I didn't go get my paper because a skunk was chewing away on my lawn right near the mailbox, and I was throwing sticks and rocks at the sonofabitch." He lost it. Words and laughter were now mixing into one sound. The story slowed to allow for the laughter. "And the fucker just looks up at me and doesn't give a shit. Goes right back to eating." I heard him sip his wine. It gurgled in his mouth, the laughter causing it to bounce in his throat. "Should have shot the bastard with salt pellets," he said. I reminded him he didn't own a gun. He ignored the logistics. "And while I'm at it, I'll let those two yappy bastard dogs next door to you have it, too. They barked all night. Pow. Pow. Salt Pellets. After a good rain, the evidence will wash away." He worked himself into a fit of laughter before hanging up to "finish his wine."

On Halloween night I answered the phone. Stacie leaned out the open front door to drop candy into the open pillowcases of aliens and cheerleaders with pink hair. Kai rocked in his bouncer, still looking surprised by the contraption's response to his most minute movements.

"I'm stuck handing out candy to these goddamn creepy bastards. Trick-or-treat bullshit," Pops said on the phone. He always hated Halloween. Every year Mom swore he wouldn't have to answer the door, smiling at kids with plastic cleavers lodged into vinyl masks. But then the phone would ring or she'd need to take a "quick" shower. She'd promise it'd only be a minute. And there my dad would stand at the front door with a basket full of candy, dropping M&Ms and Heath bars into open pillow sacks, kids begging for treats.

"And stay off my lawn when you leave," he said.

"Stop yelling at them. They're kids," I said.

"And they need to keep off my goddamn lawn." I could hear the singsong of *trick or treat* in the background. "This is the perfect time to tell every kid in the neighborhood to stay off my lawn. Especially that little shit down the street and his dopey brother. They think this is some kind of pass-through. Dumbasses. You know that kid walked around the neighborhood, cutting through lawns with a running lawnmower? Striped all our yards, then had the balls to knock on my door asking if I wanted him to mow my lawn? Dopey, I tell you."

Trick or treat.

"Be nice," I scolded. I'd removed the screen from our storm window and passed out candy to masked children at my own house. Stacie picked up Kai from the bouncer and nursed him on the couch near the window, peeking through the blinds when I called out particularly adorable outfits.

Trick or treat.

"I just don't get it," my dad continued. "Why would you want to put paint all over your face and dress up? If these kids put this sort of time and effort into something useful, I'd happily give them candy. Math, picking weeds, that should get you a reward, not dressing up like a complete idiot."

I handed more candy through the missing window.

"Worked my ass off for money and these kids are just begging for free food." Before I could reprimand him again, tell him to hush or the kids would hear, he began laughing. *That* laugh. The one that sends him into a spiral of gasps and breaths, tears rushing down his scrunched-up face, unable to stop himself even if he tried. He never tried.

"And where is your mother?" His voice raised in pitch. He'd initiated the laughter. There was no turning back. "I got this disease and I still have to hand out candy." *Breath. Breath.* "ALS? Who cares? Hand out these Snickers." *Wheeze.* His laughter was infectious. You were drawn in when he laughed. The laughter was a manifest of something unable to be seen—like a sound wave mapped out on a grid. An earthquake sketched on scrolling paper. You were mesmerized, even when you had no idea of the source.

It wouldn't be long—a few weeks, a month, before Kai would begin laughing. He's programmed for it. Genetics.

In the beginning I thought every chortle from my dad was a side effect of the disease. Fifteen to forty-five percent of ALS patients "suffer" from Pseudobulbar Affect or "emotional lability," which consists of uncontrollable laughter, crying or smiling. Patients are offered medicine to control the laughter. To fix it.

But that wasn't what rushed from my dad's belly on Halloween night. It was laughter like the time when Grandma carved a man with a penis out of an orange peel on my twentieth birthday party. Pa covered his face. Laughter leaked through. This wasn't something medical doctors could diagnose, though it was infectious. My dad pulled the pin, tossed the grenade, and let the shrapnel hit anyone within his reach. I laughed my chest into pain on the other end of the phone. We laughed a duet of breaths until our lungs forced us to pause for air. This laughter was a side effect not of disease, but of life.

Trick or treat.

"Goddamn Lou Gehrig's disease and I still have to hand out candy. A terminal disease won't even get me out of this." Children's voices rang in the background.

"Pa, stop, you're going to scare the kids."

I could hear the children saying thank you, as my old man dropped candy into their buckets.

"Isn't that what Halloween is about? Being scared?" He laughed out what was left in his belly. A few last growls of laughter. They lingered for a moment until he let out a sigh, his body assumedly falling back into his chair. "Ah, shit, kiddo," he said, resigned. "I don't know anymore. I just don't know. It's all pretty damn scary."

"I know, Pops."

"Pretty damn scary."

More kids were coming up his walk, he said. He was having a hard time holding the phone while passing out candy. His hands were failing quicker than expected. Although it had only been two months since he was diagnosed, the symptoms were beginning to fall into place. His walk was more strained and those hands, they were not obeying as much as he told them. And now the laughter wore him out.

"I'm going to go, kiddo. I love you."

"Love you."

"*Goodbye.*"

Maybe it was an accident. Maybe he didn't mean to say it. But he could never take it back. It was forever.

8. Pretend

I'd always assumed the voice from behind the shower curtain couldn't be my father's. In fact, I'd never even considered the possibility. Still too young to bathe myself, my dad scrubbed the day's dirt off my body, then set me outside the tub, pulling the solid yellow curtain closed. I'd begin toweling off, and that's when Roger would appear.

He spoke in a high-pitched voice behind the curtain, asking about my day, trains, favorite comic book characters. I ran the towel between my toes, answering his questions, explaining how Batman was superior to the others because he was just a man who did super acts without super powers. I told Roger how I wanted a skateboard for Christmas, that I'd someday marry my neighbor Carrie, how I was scared of full moons, wished all popsicles were lemon.

Roger listened. He'd laugh at my stories, but never divulged much about himself. Never revealed what kind of car he drove, if he had any vacations planned, his favorite time of year. Though, in all fairness, I probably never asked.

Aside from listening to my stories, Roger would sing. When I ran out of tales each day, Roger would bellow from the other side of the curtain. He'd sing Led Zeppelin and Hendrix. I'd sing along, off pitch. Like two fools, Roger and I mastered the classic rock canon. I'd hum the guitars, buzzing my lips against my teeth, while Roger tapped out the drum solos for "Wipeout" and "Moby Dick" against the curtain. I'd sit on the closed toilet, tapping my toes in the tiny puddles pooling on the bathroom floor. Whenever he finished, Roger's fingers left wet imprints on the curtain, marking the beats, marking where he'd been.

"I just thought it would be fun while you waited for me," my dad said. His face contorted, cheeks filled in like he was smiling, but eyes stretched down with remorse. I'd just asked for Roger, and my dad said, "You know he's not real, right?" I wedged myself between the toilet and the vanity cabinet. The porcelain toilet bowl was cold on my ribs. I sobbed, heaved, tears that made my back tremor.

My dad stood naked, the curtain open, soap creeping down his side. He tried explaining that he was just pretending to be Roger, thought I knew. Like Santa Claus or the Tooth Fairy. He said I was old enough to know by now. He attempted to say "I'm sorry" so many times. But I wouldn't let him finish. When he began the apology, I kicked my feet against the tub, heels thudding against the sides, legs rigid. I wanted to leave dents, wanted to kick the tub in, make it cave into itself. I kicked away each apology, each attempt to make it right. Bring him back. I didn't want words. I wanted Roger. But instead I had my father, standing before me, drenched, and silenced by my fits.

I told him I didn't believe him. That Roger had just gone away, that he was real. I shrieked. My tears now mixed with the water from my hair running down my temples.

Mom stood in the doorway. Her two naked boys deadlocked, separated by the tub. She said it would be okay, trying to wrap the towel around my body. But I fought her too. I kicked and screamed and.

"Mike."

I looked at my father. His mouth. Where the words came from. But the words weren't my father's. The voice was higher. It was Roger's voice softly being spoken from my dad's lips.

"See?" he said. "It's been me all along."

He switched back to his real voice. "I thought you knew that it's always been me. The two of us. We don't need Roger. We can get along without him."

I stared, shivering, now aware of the absence.

I stood up.

Allowed Mom to wrap me in the towel.

My lower lip still quivered when I breathed in the short breaths. Between starts and stops of tears I said, "But I never said goodbye."

My dad closed the shower curtain. The faucet squeaked as he turned it. The pipes moaned, paused and the water began tapping against the bathtub floor. The voice inside the tub cleared his throat. Roger said, "It's okay, Michael. I'll miss you, but your dad will take good care of you. Always."

I didn't say anything. Mom squeezed my shoulder. She asked if I wanted to say goodbye. I shook my head. Because I knew Roger was already gone. How do you say goodbye to the dead, even when they're standing before you?

Mom ushered me out of the room, her arm around my shoulder.

As we left, I listened to the body moving inside the shower, movement detected by shifts in patterns—water striking the wall, curtain, floor. Like Daredevil, the blind superhero who could see through sound, I imagined movement, the twisting of the body. I tried to imagine Roger's final movements, but could only see my dad, upright, naked, rinsing the remaining soap that clung to his body. Water sprayed the curtain, leaving behind trails of where he'd been.

9. Paper Roses

Mom called it two months before my dad's first appointment. Before the tests. Before the first office visit with the GP who delivered the news, said he wasn't sure, only a guess, but it seemed to be. Mom could have been a medical researcher. She's been distrustful of the medical community since she was sixteen and her mother went in for an ulcer and didn't come out. Since her OB-GYN left some of the placenta inside. Since her step-mom voluntarily underwent preventative cancer surgery—went in without cancer, came out with cancer. Dead within two years. Since she realized it's their job. *A* job. Something they can leave behind at the end of the day before returning to life.

After the doctors confirmed the disease Mom sat on the couch each night, her laptop making her face glow, searching for cures—tiny scraps of hope. After their first visit with the ALS experts, Pa was given a prescription for Rilutek, which only offered a few extra months tacked on at the end. When it was at its worst. Other than that, the doctors said the best Pa could do was sign up for experiments with their researchers. The clinic only offered one—mega doses of antibiotics. They said it almost certainly wasn't a cure, but they were just curious. My parents declined that experiment.

Mom checked into her evening job like clockwork. 6:30 PM. While my dad watched the world news from his recliner, the only chair to survive the living room redecoration, the soundtrack of flooding and war and famine and disease played in the background while she punched combinations of words into her computer. *ALS cures experimental drugs therapies acupuncture diet herbs medicines genes genetic. Stem. Cells.*

George W. Bush, the president at that time, banned federal funding for stem cell research. He said he was protecting human life. Didn't want to compromise a breath. The forums, the experts, the medical journals, and the hopeful thought the answer lay in stem cell replacement. But without the government there wasn't enough money for research. Or time left for my dad.

Pa told Mom to stop. Let it go. There was nothing she could do. But she wouldn't. Any time we'd stop by, Kai in tow, she'd remove her glasses and put her computer to sleep, but never off. She'd make up for the hour when we left.

One night I looked through our back kitchen window at 7 PM and noticed a light on in the back of my parents' house. Mom converted my old bedroom into a "project room" that housed a large wooden table and her sewing machine. I could see Mom standing by the window, looking down at the table, her shoulders and hands moving. I called.

"You know it's past seven, right?" I said.

"What's your point?" she asked.

"You're supposed to be researching." The hope Mom's research offered extended well beyond herself. Stacie and I both felt that as long as she looked, there was reason to believe. She'd found leads on suggested diets, stem cell replacement in Mexico, a doctor in Korea who might have the drug. There were nights when she cried, gushing in my dad's arms, because she worried the high protein diet she read about made it worse. But she picked herself up and tried again. If she stopped, there was nothing left because his doctors weren't pining away. It was over for them. But not for Mom.

"I can see you through the window," I said.

She laughed and flicked me off. "Can you see this?"

"Get back to work, woman," I said. "This disease isn't going to cure itself."

"I'm tired of it. It's the same thing every night. No answers, just guesses." She'd hooked up with several people on the ALS forums, knowing the folks by their handles, codenames like the CB my dad used on vacations. "Breaker breaker 1-9, this is Red Turtle, how 'bout ya Harley, you got a copy?" Mom followed the posts of "Eddie Spaghetti," a man with ALS who fed news to the forums. He posted jokes when he had his down days, and let his followers know his wife, his caregiver, was losing it. She'd been talking about leaving him because it was too much for her.

She breathed. "So I'm making flowers instead."

Roses. Paper Roses. For two weeks straight at 6:30 PM Mom's back light flicked on, and she folded strips of paper into perfect replicas of roses. Some bloomed open, while others in the bouquet remained tightly shut, folded into themselves. I'd check on the light periodically, and after an hour, it flicked off. She followed the same routine for nearly two weeks. Then she stopped.

She returned to the couch, researching well into the *Seinfeld* reruns that Pa lost himself in. She looked for the perfect combination of keywords, the password that would unlock a cure while the bouquet of a dozen paper roses sat in a vase in the project room, unwilting, perfect, never decaying or dying, until enough sun shone through the window tinting each white rose a worn shade of yellow.

10. Canings

Six months after being diagnosed my dad relied entirely on a cane to support his weakening body. After winter break he agreed to take it to work—until that point he casually leaned on walls and held onto computer carts in the halls to mask the disease. My dad always showed up to work hours before he was supposed to. He said it was during the quiet, before teachers and students arrived, that he could catch up and get his work done. Even though he wasn't compensated for that time, he said it was worth it. He'd turn on computer labs and check servers before service tickets came streaming into his office.

The first day back after winter break John, the shop teacher, happened to arrive at the same hour as my dad. John saw him walking down the hall, his cane pulling his body forward. "What did you do?" John shouted down the hall. Dad said his voice echoed in the empty corridor. "Rough break? Screw up your back lifting that grandson of yours around? You're falling apart, old man."

It was hard for Pa to walk and speak at the same time. All of his energy needed to be concentrated on one activity. He said he paused in the hallway, leaned against the wall, and waited for John to reach him—all the while shouting about growing old. By the time he reached him, my dad recovered. And then he told him. My dad never padded his words. When I was eight and fell off my skateboard, painting my face with asphalt, my dad said, "That's what your hands are for." That day in the hallway, I'm sure he delivered the news of his disease much in the same manner. Pa said John acted like he didn't know what to say. Lots of apologies about the disease and the old-age quips. Pa told him to forget about it and asked that he not say anything because he wasn't ready to quit his job because he needed the money; he wanted Mom to be taken care of. And even more, I believe he needed to know he was still able to wake up every morning and move. John assured him he'd keep it quiet.

Pa said by the end of the day there were more bodies in his office than service tickets. People gave him *the* eyes he always said he avoided. His best friend David Lackey, the head of the English Department, stopped by. Shook his hand. Said he'd be there every step of the way.

As the weeks went on, my dad upgraded his cane to one that opened into a seat—when walking the halls of work became too tiresome, he could rest, gather enough energy to finish. I only saw my dad use his cane in the confines of his home to get from the living room to the kitchen. It wasn't until early March that I accidentally ran into my parents at the grocery store. I was parking my car when I saw my mother and father walking across the parking lot. His movement was so slow, labored by shortness of breath and failing muscle. Until that moment the disease was contained, at least in my mind, to his house. I'd never witnessed this walk in the light of day from a man whose strength was unparalleled. My dad once relocated a telephone pole across the yard by himself. He rode marathon bike rides. He cherished physical labor and movement above all else.

As soon as the sliding grocery store doors opened, my dad latched onto the shopping cart, hung his cane on the handle, and his walk immediately returned to normal. He was able to hide it all behind the wheels and support of the cart. But that walk couldn't be returned. Those steps became something concrete for me. I never went into the store to shop that day. Instead, I returned home, lifted my son out of his bouncer, and pulled him to my chest while I cried into my wife's shoulder.

The living room was entirely dark, save the TV, which flickered bursts of light on my dad's skeletal face. His BiPAP breathed. When I entered the front door, he nodded slightly, blinking both eyes hello. Mom lay on the couch, curled small beneath Big Brown, the name she gave to my childhood blanket. Her face was wet. She wiped her face on the blanket. Heaved as she cried. I set the bag of bagels on the kitchen table and then sat on the couch across from my dad. Mom held me. And we cried together.

Pa shook his head and mouthed *stop* through his mask. Colors of light bounced off the windows, walls. Pa slowly raised his only working hand to the mask and tapped it, nodding to Mom.

"Switch it?" she asked. He nodded.

Mom pulled the full face mask off and replaced it with a nose unit that didn't offer nearly as much air, but allowed my dad to speak without being encumbered by the plastic mask. When he wore the full mask, the lack of language made him even more distant.

His words were whispers. Mom shut off the TV then clicked on a small corner lamp. She curled back into herself.

"This is a good thing," Pa whispered. His language was slow. "I can't. I can't live anymore like this." Then he began his list. He said, "Can't sleep, can't breathe, can't move, can't even shit. And there are no more movies, I watched them all."

Some drool came out of his mouth. He couldn't laugh, his body lacked the muscle, but he paused, his tongue slipping from his mouth, a silent laugh. "It will get better," he said. "I'll miss you and Stacie and Kai and Mom." He said every name, even though speaking was wearing him down. He said every damn name.

His face was barely visible between my tears. He straightened the mask with his working hand. Air whooshed out as the seal with his nose was broken. The machine screamed a warning. Pa resealed the connection and gasped.

"This is fucking insane," he said. All his words were gapped by breaths. "I need to go. I love you. I love you. This isn't you two. It's just misery. Life is misery."

Mom heaved. She reached for my hand. Squeezed when I broke.

This chair my father was sitting in had been his home for nearly a year. The only piece of furniture he could find some comfort in. They'd tried a half-dozen wheel chairs, some with electronic lifts and adjustments. But this reclining chair in the living room was it. My dad sat there for a year, unable to walk. Unable to leave the house. Only lifted and hoisted by Mom to use the portable toilet and be wheeled into bed.

I suggested food—told Mom she needed to eat to make it through the day. She said not now, that she couldn't. My dad hadn't eaten in days. Now he couldn't even swallow liquid. No more muscle. Water was too thick.

"What if there is something else?" I asked. "What if something is coming soon. Maybe some hope for a cure."

Pa closed his eyes. "Do this for me," he said. "It's all I ask. I love you all. Do this for me. Because I waited too long, and now I can't."

11. Who's Joe?

Pa waved his cane wildly in the power equipment store. "Joe? Who's Joe? Are you Joe?" I looked at Mom and she shook her head.

The man behind the counter straightened his baseball hat. "He's out back—I can get him." Pa nodded his head, put his cane back on the ground, took a deep breath. "Who should I tell him is..."

"Tell him it's Dan Hemery," Pa said, panting. "Tell Joe it's Dan Hemery."

The man nodded and went out the back door to call Joe.

Pa worked his way to the large commercial mowers in the back of the showroom—past the blowers and weed whackers. Pa's gait was awkward, as if he had to heave each leg forward to walk. He pushed on the deck of a large, red, zero-turn mower with his cane, tapping the wheels. "Something like this should do."

"'Where's Jooooe?'" I said, waving an imaginary cane around. Mom laughed and looked at Pa.

"What?" he asked.

"What was with the cane waving? 'Jooooe, where's Joe?'"

Mom leaned against a mower and now began laughing harder than before. My dad smirked. "What? I just want to get this taken care of quickly."

"You're not going to start using that *thing*," Mom pointed to the cane, "like some sort of old man."

"'Joooooooe,'" I said.

Pa lifted his hand not on the cane and flicked me off, laughed, and backed himself against a mower for support.

After the winter thaw, first rains, and some sun, Stacie, Kai, and I drove past my parents' house to find my dad sitting on a milk crate at the top of the lawn, his mower idling in front of him. We pulled in as Pa stood, engaged the blades and walked a stripe to the bottom of the yard, slowly turned, and mowed another back. He moved the crate. Sat again, chest heaving for air. Stacie remained in the car while I walked to Pa to see if he was okay.

"I'll mow your yard for you," I said.

Pa shook his head. "I need to know. I have to do it once this year so I know."

"How long have you been out here?"

"An hour."

The front was only half done and he hadn't even touched the back. It typically took an hour to mow the entire half-acre. "I can only support myself for one stripe down and back."

I told him I'd finish the yard, send Stacie home with Kai. But he shook his head. "Just once. I'll have to justify it in my head later. I'll need to know when I absolutely have to call it quits." He reached out, grabbed my hand and held it. His hands were cold. It was early in the season, and like all the previous years, he was the first mow in the neighborhood. Dandelions hadn't even begun to show themselves.

He used my hand for support, closed his eyes, and pulled himself upright. I asked him if he was sure. He nodded. "Thirty more stripes or so." He engaged the blades. "I should be done before dark."

Joe was a soft-spoken man who waited for my dad to switch his cane to his left hand so they could shake. Joe said he knew of my dad from

Bob, one of my dad's former employees when he was the head janitor of an elementary school. Bob sometimes gave my dad hell as an employee—pushing back when Pa said the job wasn't done well enough. Bob organized silent protests when my dad brought in donuts for the crew, refusing to eat the food because he thought my dad worked them too hard. But when he found out about my dad's illness, he called my mom. It had been years since my dad and he worked together—my dad moved on to be hired as the head computer technician for the school district and Bob, ironically enough, was head of maintenance for the schools. He told Mom that my dad taught him everything. He said he never had a father of his own, so he fought my dad's "fatherly" ways. But, he said, no one ever taught him to work hard, earn his money like a man, except my dad. He owed him everything, he said.

Joe supplied mowers to the school and Bob told him to cut my dad a deal on the mower. He explained that this would be his lifeline for a year—allow him to be in control of his yard as his body decayed. Joe listened to my dad with a quiet reverence. My dad told me to sit on the mower and suggested Mom give it a try. Mom said she didn't want to, but he insisted. He said, "Eventually you'll have to mow the yard when this kills me." He looked at Joe and said, "Will she be able to handle this thing?" Mom wiped her tears into her sleeve as she sat on the mower.

Joe nodded and said, "Yes, but we need to make sure this works for you, too."

"I don't know how long I'll even be able to walk," Pa said. "So, I have to know if she can handle it."

"She can," Joe said. "Do you feel strong enough to walk to the shop out back and try it out? We can make sure it works for you."

My dad nodded. Gripping his cane, the four of us took the slow walk through the shop where mowers were hoisted up on lifts and parts were stacked in crates. The trial mowers were at the bottom of a pitched gravel drive. "Can you do it?" I asked Pa. He nodded and took careful step after careful step down the gravel. Joe walked ahead of us, giving my dad his dignity, to get the mower prepped and pull it as close to my dad as possible. I reached for my dad's elbow and he shook his head. Instead I walked just behind him, ready to catch him, just in case.

When we reached the mower Joe explained how to get on it. There was usually a rubber stomp pad, but it had worn off. Joe stepped up on the mower twice, showing the best approach. My dad nodded and handed Mom his cane. He gripped the handle with his right hand and put his right leg where the stomp pad should be. As he leaned forward to grip the casing of the mower with his left hand, his leg slipped on the slick metal mowing deck. The movement was awkward, and with less muscle, he was unable to compensate, so his body lunged forward toward the mower.

I'd been shadowing his every move as he approached the machine and the moment his body flinched, I wrapped my arms around his waist and pulled him hard to my body. I held him there for a moment. He was skinnier than four months ago. I could feel his bones against my chest as we breathed together.

Mom rushed in and put the cane in his hand, and Joe helped to right him. My dad opened his cane into the stool and sat, breathing in and out. Joe said nothing, but walked to the machine and worked the toe of his boot over the metal step. "It's slippery. I should have dried it more. I'm so sorry."

My dad shook his head and waved his hand. Unable to speak he just breathed for what felt like an eternity. I checked to see if any of the workers had seen. My father's pride was strong. This disease was weakness and he never tolerated his own weakness, physical or mental. The workers hadn't noticed, but surely they might see something was off, the four of us standing around this running mower.

"Let me have a go at it," I said. My dad looked up at me, his eyes unblinking. "I mean, you'll be riding it most of the time, but I'll be damned if I'm going to push mow my yard anymore. If we have this beast I'll be using it, so let me see how she feels."

My dad nodded. "That would be good," he said. His breaths turned into a smile. "That would be good."

I climbed up on the mower. The deck was slippery. His body could not have compensated for the shift without the rubber pad. Joe pulled the handles in and told me to put my hands on them. I misheard his instructions and put my hands on his hands, which still gripped the handles. He didn't react, but went with it, showing me how to turn the mower and move it forward. I could hear my dad laughing from his stool. "Why are you holding his hands?" he asked. His cheeks were red with laughter.

"I wasn't going to say anything, but I wondered the same thing," Joe said, laughing.

Mom rubbed Pa's back, and the workers up the hill carried on with their tasks, ignoring the seemingly normal moment of laughter.

I took the mower for a spin, enjoying the crispness of the turns. The machine reacted to the slightest shift of the finger. It provided control. Power. And movement. This, for my father, would be the extension of his body that he craved. He'd buy the machine and it would provide movement for my dad for an entire year. He'd even mow my lawn some days, before sitting became a chore.

Mom decided not to try it out. She said she trusted my judgment. We eventually worked our way back up the gravel incline and into the showroom, where we found Bob waiting.

"Hot damn, Hemery," he said when we walked in. "You'll be able to wax the piss out of this machine. Did you see all the metal on it?"

Pa shook his head. His eyes were tired. But he never opened his stool. Instead he leaned on the mower's roll bar for support—refusing to sit because he surely needed to stand and talk like men talk. Upright. Eye to eye. Sitting was weakness.

Bob shook my dad's hand and hugged my mom. "What do you think?" Pa asked.

"This is the one to get," he said. Bob looked at Joe and said, "Can you get him a better seat? This one is shit. And a seatbelt?" I'd forgotten that my dad would need that support soon—a restraint to keep him upright. "And don't go charging them more, I know you have that shit just sitting in the back room." Joe said of course and worked up the paperwork for the mower.

Pa and Bob talked about work, the mower, anything but the disease. Bob teased my dad about his need for perfection. And Pa called him a lazy sonofabitch. We laughed about Pa waving his cane and shouting, "Where's Joe?" And we laughed when Bob admitted he had work to do, but decided to come check out the mower instead. "Just wanted to make sure you weren't going cheap and buying some residential-grade shit." We all knew he came to make sure Joe cut us a much lower price. And to thank my dad for being a dad to him by helping us laugh our way out of ourselves.

12. Done

I was washing the back windshield of my car, soap suds slipping down the trunk, when Pa pulled in our driveway. He was still able to drive—enough muscle to accelerate, stop, and turn—machines gave him more life than he'd otherwise have. When he bought the Civic hybrid two years before the symptoms, he asked my opinion. "It's the responsible thing to do for the environment. Right?" he asked. If he took care of it right, it might be the last car he'd buy—get him through retirement. It would be the last car he'd buy.

"That's it," he said, leaning out his window.

I dropped the washrag into the soap bucket. "Well, how's it feel?" I knew how it felt, so I don't know why I asked. Forced retirement because of a terminal disease felt like a miniature death. My dad planned to work well into his seventies. He thrived off work—loved the routine. The business. He would have let Mom retire first, soon, and then work until he couldn't stand it anymore. Now he couldn't stand anymore.

He and Mom decided Spring Break would be the natural breaking point. He'd leave and not return—run out the hundreds of sick days, serve as a consultant and then officially retire. The school was frantic because he ran the technology for eight schools: the network and the individual computers. He was the technological heart and brains of the entire district. They hired an interim replacement to shadow him for weeks, but she was overwhelmed by his workload. She said there needed to be more hires to fill his vacancy. Other districts hired at least three people to do his job.

"It feels weird," he said. "Not just because of the circumstances. It just feels strange to know I won't go back tomorrow. Ever."

"Were they nice? Big send off?"

"You know how it is. Everyone is pretty busy. Bob picked me up in his Hummer and we went to lunch." It turns out the sendoff was bigger than that. Nearly every staff member in the district wrote him a note and one of the teachers tied them all together with yarn. The final product was the size of a bowling ball and maybe nearly as heavy. People thanked him for his patience, his kindness, his knowledge, his dedication. Mom said he later admitted that his office was filled with streams of people hugging him, thanking him, promising this wasn't the end of their relationships. Tears upon tears upon tears.

"What's it like inside a Hummer?" I asked.

"Pretty cool. Big. It was cool."

Pa flicked his nail on the steering wheel.

"You going to be okay?"

"It's so fucked up." Pa sighed. "Just not the plan at all. Your mom is going to have to keep working now. She's worked enough."

"You can't control any of this." He nodded. "Maybe just enjoy some time off for the first time in your life. Spend time with Kai." While you can.

He nodded. "I'll let you work. You missed a spot," he said, pointing to the smear of mud on the back bumper.

I laughed. "Disease can't stop your devotion to perfection and detail."

He shook his head. I leaned in and kissed his cheek. He said he loved me. I loved him.

"Tomorrow is the beginning of a new phase," I said. "We'll be okay. Maybe it will even be good."

Pa gagged on air. His tongue protracted and his torso cocked forward. Mom rushed to his side. There was no stomach muscle left to cough. The only movement left was his tongue, face, right arm, and a slight flinch in the two fingers of his right hand. The rest was frozen. His brain stopped communicating with the body, except for an occasional trickle to an extremity. He was all skeleton, bone jutting out of flesh.

"Mom," I said, "what should I do?"

She didn't answer, but leapt to his side to thrust him upright. She pulled the nose adapter out with one hand and reconnected the full facial mask for more air.

"Mom."

Pa's eyes widened. He tapped the mask with his functional hand. His eyes bulged. The machine shrieked because the seal was broken.

"Mom, what do I do?"

"Nothing," she said. "Nothing. There is nothing. Nothing."

She pulled off the mask. Pa's tongue came out. Another silent gag. She reconnected the mask.

"Mom."

The machine silenced. The seal latched that time. My dad's eyes closed. His chest moved in and out. Mom pulled his fleece blanket over him. The air made him cold. He was always covered because he lacked the muscle to shiver, to create heat. Mom sewed him a fleece blanket with frogs on the outside. Mom's cousin Jim called Pa a "frog" when they first met because he was from France. When Jim introduced Pa to Mom, he said this was his "froggy friend, Dan." My dad took it in stride because he was thrilled to have new friends in America. The word remained a joke in the family ever since. Inside the blanket were dozens of "hugs," the word embroidered over and over. She said the blanket would keep him warm and remind him she was always holding him, since her touch, any touch, caused his body great agony. Simple blankets and sheets at bedtime hurt his body because of their weight. So when he sat in his chair, for some reason, this blanket enveloped him perfectly and painlessly.

"Mom."

She was all tears, kneeling before my dad, clutching his chest. She'd bathed him, moved his body for him, fed him. And this was the end. She moaned into his chest, then let out a sound like a high-pitched scream.

Mom.

Pa opened his eyes. Looked down at her. Shut them again.

13. Napa

If he wasn't dying, they never would have taken the trip. Too much money. Time. It involved flying, which Mom dreaded. But when Mom's sister said she was surprising my uncle with the trip to Napa for his sixtieth birthday and asked if Mom and Pa wanted to accompany them, they didn't hesitate and booked the trip for Spring Break.

The major anxiety for my folks revolved around how to navigate the airports. Pa couldn't walk more than thirty feet and now relied on his cane anytime he was upright. They'd face security checkpoints, the removal of shoes, long journeys to the gate, and boarding and unboarding the planes. But Mom said they'd figure it out. She made calls, advance arrangements with the airline and airports: shuttles and assistance from all who would provide it. It was worth it, she said. "We need this."

Pa called from the first boarding gate.

"Good people work here in Cleveland," he said. "They didn't make me walk through the checkpoint, but used one of those handheld detectors while I sat in the wheelchair *they* provided. So nice. Lots of 'enjoy your trips' and just all around kindness." He said a shuttle was waiting for them at the security checkpoint and deposited all four of them right at the gate. "I felt like a celebrity."

Pa never accepted charity or special treatment, so this kind of attention would typically embarrass him. But he must have known there were no other options and seemed to embrace the support. There was nothing else he could do, so he permitted his disease to make him feel like a rock star.

Stacie and I received daily phone calls, status updates. They hooked up with my mom's cousin, Jim, who lived in San Francisco, the guy who introduced Mom to my dad when she was only fourteen. They committed their mornings to sightseeing, and their afternoons belonged to various wineries in the valley, taking train tours, eating at five-star restaurants, and drinking enough to forget why they were there.

"It's all just so beautiful," Pa said. I received the call while changing Kai's diaper. He cooed on the changing table.

"What's that, Pops?" I asked.

"This whole place. The whole thing. It's just gorgeous. It's so nice here. Like, heaven. Flowers. The temperature is nice. The wine is nice. It smells nice. The rows and rows of vines, all perfectly lined up and ordered, stretching out forever. I could just sit here and watch them…" He trailed off.

"You drunk?" I asked.

My dad giggled a bit.

"Where is everyone else? They with you?"

"No, your mom and them went for a walk around the property of this vineyard, but I said I'd just sit here on this bench and finish this bottle of wine because what the hell, you know?" He laughed again. "I wish you could see this place. The weather has been perfect. They say it's all going to turn to heat in a week or so and get miserable, but right now, right now it's the best. I'm so happy just sitting here and the wine, oh the wine, it's good. We just ordered a case to be shipped home. You'll have to try it."

I wanted to ask how he was navigating the terrain, even the parking lots. He had to be doing more walking on this trip than he'd done in some time. And I wondered if it was killing him not to walk more. Typically on vacations he and Mom would be up well before the sun to explore and traverse trails. They were never content resting in one place too long. But I knew this was different, and I wanted to ask how he was dealing with that drastic change. But it would have been unfair to pull him out of that moment, that blissful, euphoric moment of peace.

"Good thing that beautiful kid of yours is back at home, otherwise I might just stay here, at this vineyard forever."

"Thanks, Pops, we're not good enough?"

He laughed. "You know what I mean." I could hear him sipping his wine. "I think I'm drunk. We just spent way too much on wine, like $500. We don't have that kind of money to blow on wine, but they're shipping it for a buck. But it's good. So beautiful here." He laughed and laughed.

I can only recall one prior occasion when my dad got really sauced. I was in high school, and after cleaning the house windows on a muggy day he worked down several beers, forgetting Mom's friends were coming over for dinner. I happened upon him holding his head in his bedroom on the edge of his bed. When I walked in he started laughing uncontrollably and told me to sit next to him. "I'm so fucked up," he said, laughing. I told him that it was okay, but I had to adjust to this version of my dad because I'd never really seen him drunk. "And I forgot your mom's friends were coming over. Are they here?" I said yes. "Oh man, she's going to be so pissed." He talked this way for some time until his laughter turned to tears and he pronounced how much he loved me and Mom. We were his world, he said, all he ever cared about.

Now I heard him sigh on the phone. "I'm telling you kid, I miss you, but I could stay right here forever. Just beautiful."

We talked for several more minutes, while I slipped Kai's blue baseball shirt over his head and placed him on his play mat. Pa spoke about their train ride, and Cousin Jim, unaware at that time that he'd be next to go; even then the cancer was crowding Jim's insides. Pa said he loved me, to kiss Stacie and Kai for him. He said the word "beautiful" at least a dozen more times before saying, "See you soon, if we decide to come back."

The remainder of their trip was equally as delightful—winery after winery, perfect day after perfect day. "Despite it all," Mom said when she called one night, "this is one of the best vacations we've ever had."

Their return trek rocked them back into reality more quickly than they would have preferred. The people at LAX weren't as empathetic as the workers at the Cleveland airport. Despite calling ahead, security insisted my dad remove his shoes. Said he had to walk through the checkpoint without his cane. Mom said my dad pleaded, then fumed, but they were rigid with their rules. So he staggered through, gripping the plastic walls of the machine to just get through. This was a man who never exhibited weakness, physical or mental, and those motherfuckers at the airport left him out there for all to see. They let his failing muscles drag his body through that machine. Mom was waiting for him on the other side with a wheelchair, and she said he collapsed into it, drained from the ordeal. There were no trams, no shuttles, and the official Mom spoke to explained that even if you call ahead there are no guarantees. "There are too many people passing through this place to take care of individuals," he said. So she pushed him in the wheelchair to their gate. On display. When they finally arrived at the gate she asked if he wanted to call me, just to chat, but he said he was too winded. He said he needed to rest, to figure out how he was going to walk onto the plane and come home.

14. Wine and Guitars

"Wine and guitars: they can cure anything,
even if only for a while."
—David Lackey

Pa's friendship with David began at the high school where they both worked. "He never acts like he's better than anyone else," Pa said about David when he first mentioned his name. "Sometimes teachers get their degrees and think they're better than you. But not David—he gets it." David, or Mr. Lackey, taught at the high school I attended. I had his wife, Linda, for a few classes, but never David—he taught the honors courses, and I wasn't interested in English enough at the time to pursue those classes. He and my dad would engage in transitory talks about motorcycles and music while my dad installed updates on his computer. They arranged some dinners to include their wives, and soon the Lackeys became a staple in my parents' lives, sharing bottles of wine after school and exchanging gifts on the holidays.

Though they had much in common, David and my dad really bonded over guitars. Just a few years before the diagnosis my dad bought a new guitar—a Fender Stratocaster to replace his "piece of shit" Gretsch guitar he played when he was a teenager. He gave his old one to David's son. "As a collector's item," he told me. "Not to play. That guitar never sounded right." After enough drinks at the Lackeys' parties, Pa and David would end up with guitars in hands playing a few chords for their wives. But Pa was also self-conscious of his talents, too reserved to really play in front of people. He believed in perfection above all else, so until he achieved flawlessness, he never really let loose.

Mom also took an interest in learning to play later in life, so the two of them would jam after work in the basement, learning chords and then songs. It didn't take long for my dad to work up the chops he had when he was a teenager. But instead of "Sergeant Pepper" and "Louie Louie," Pa now found a connection with the blues—the long sustained chords of Gary Moore and Buddy Guy would resonate from the basement. Although Mom said she liked to play, her interest seemed to wane, so Pa would spend time each night with his guitar alone in the basement, making it cry.

Pa rarely indulged in doing things just to make himself happy. He claimed there was always a lawn to mow, gutters to clean. He was perpetual motion. But he told me he found much pleasure in playing again. He practiced with the same fervor he brought to everything in his life and strove for perfection. When I'd visit Mom, I'd hear him in the basement playing the same run over and over until it was smooth. She said he'd manically play like that for hours. He'd never move on until he got each part right. When he'd emerge from the basement he'd smile in a way he rarely did—it was as if he viewed playing as some sort of guilty pleasure of gluttony, and for one of the first times in his life, he celebrated it.

For the annual family holiday soirée (a stress-free event Stacie and I hosted two weeks before Christmas for the family members who had to cook and clean for the *real* holidays), Mom and Pa would perform a concert for the guests, typically a range of Christmas tunes. Mom always had her nose buried in the sheet music as she was taxed to hit the notes, while Pa would shake his head and laugh as Mom rummaged through the songs.

For the last soirée, the one before his diagnosis, Pa performed a song after the two of them finished with the Christmas melodies "Jingle Bells" and "O Come All Ye Faithful." He'd been practicing it for months, he said. He apologized in advance if he messed up. But then he lowered his head, turned up the amp, and let the guitar sing. I knew my old man could play, but I never knew he could play like *that.* In high school, when I took up the drums, he'd play "Wipe Out" and some other rock standards with me in the basement. But that performance in my living room was something else. It was music. It was years of frustration from being overworked and underpaid spilling out of his fingers onto the fret board. No one at the party blinked. My mom's cousin Jim, who used to play in a band with my dad when they were teens, closed his eyes during the performance and swayed forward and back. Pa never looked up once during the song. When his eyes were open, they were following his fingers up and down the neck of the guitar. They moved effortlessly. Note after note after note. A trance. A translation.

When he finished, he looked up, we clapped, and he blew on his fingers. Humble and never able to celebrate his own gifts, Pa shook his head and said, "Fingers don't work like they did when I was younger." Of course, no one knew. And if he would have known, he never would have played. Months later a therapist told him he should continue playing. She said that the movement would help keep Pa's hand muscles strong, and maybe even allow them to move a little bit longer than they would otherwise.

But he never did. Pa and Mom would go to the Lackeys' house for many more dinners and even more bottles of wine. Each time David would ask my dad to play. He had a basement of guitars, some he'd bought and some he'd made. He knew about the therapist's suggestion. "Who cares how it sounds?" he'd say. "Let's just make them wail. No rock 'n roll. Just the blues. The slow, screaming blues." Even after the alcohol saturated my dad's breath, he'd decline the offer.

The Lackeys would be there until the end. They'd come with bottles of wine even when Pa's throat could no longer swallow much more than water. Wine ran too thick, causing him to choke. They came even when Pa said he was too tired to have company. And every time after they left Pa would always say how pleased he was they insisted. He said, "When they're here I forget about myself for a while. I get lost in their stories."

Once when I stopped by, closer to the end, David showed my dad his latest home-made guitar. Pa laughed through his breathing mask, then asked Mom to remove it so he could say, "Sounds worse than my old damn guitar." But that was as close to the music as Pa could get. For some reason listening to music made him ill. Any kind of music now turned his stomach, he said. I believe the music used to be a direct line to my dad's emotions, the chords his voice, but the blues had already crept into my dad's arms, encapsulated his neurons, claimed his feet. That evening of the soirée at my house was his final performance. He'd never play again. Surely, it was difficult enough to see and feel the decay; he didn't need to hear it, too.

15. Taken Care Of

The doctors were entirely worthless. Every month or so my parents would drive to downtown Cleveland so a specialist could measure breaths and test muscle loss. These doctors never offered solutions, advice, or ideas for how to make any of it more tolerable or comfortable. Instead, they collected numbers so they knew how much worse it had gotten. "I don't understand what the point is," Pa said to me before a visit. "Yes, it's worse each month. It's not going to get better. Why do we have to go down there?"

"I'm sure they're just keeping track," I said.

"For themselves," Pa said. "Not for me. They're keeping numbers for their long-term research. I don't have long term. They don't give a damn about how scary this is or how I'm going to get in and out of the shower soon. They have nothing but meaningless numbers."

After the tests Pa had to meet with therapists and psychologists. "Do you feel like harming yourself?" Pa's doctor asked him one day.

He looked up at her and grinned. "Every goddamn day."

Since he retired, while Mom looked for cures, my old man tried to find the quickest way to off himself. He said he knew how this was going to end—slowly, painfully, and a burden on Mom. He said he didn't want that to happen, that he'd take care of it before things grew really bad.

"Shouldn't have bought that hybrid car," Pa said on the phone to me one afternoon. I was just finishing the dishes.

"Why?"

"Engine shuts off if you don't have your foot on the gas. Can't kill myself if the engine keeps shutting off."

"That's sick, Pa."

He laughed. "It's the truth," he said.

"Doesn't matter anyhow because of the government," Pa said. "The government won't even let me kill myself. They regulated the cars with these catalytic converters, and so I can't just close my eyes in the garage and go to sleep."

"A Cadillac converter?"

"Catalytic," Pa said and then began laughing. "Have I taught you nothing?" He began laughing even harder.

He went on to explain how the toxic emissions from cars are converted into clean air and you can't kill yourself by running the car in the garage anymore. "The mower doesn't have one, but I don't think there is enough 'oomph' to fill the whole garage with fumes. I'd probably just run out of gas and be sitting on that damn thing all afternoon." He began laughing again. "Can you imagine? Me sitting my ass on that mower and getting caught by your mother? She'd be so pissed."

"This is dark, Pa."

"Awww, lighten up," he said. "I'm not killing myself yet. Mostly because I can't figure out how to. Can't shoot myself—too messy. You know how I feel about messes."

Over the next few weeks Pa immersed himself in research. There was a "suicide vacation" he could take to Switzerland where euthanasia was legal—PBS ran a documentary called *The Suicide Tourist* about a guy with ALS who made that decision, who would go "with dignity," not allowing the disease to win. People paid money for the trip, the service, and that was that. "I've always wanted to go to Switzerland," he said.

"Stop it," Mom said, all of us in the living room. Kai was nestled in his lap, looking out the window. "So I just fly home by myself?"

"Everyone could go. You could go snowboarding," Pa said to me.

"Just stop this sort of talk."

"Kevorkian is a saint. A saint, I tell you. None of those bureaucratic assholes have any idea what it's like. I'll be damned if I'll get entombed. Scares the heck out of me. Think about it; I won't be able to move a thing except my eyes. My eyes. That is not life. That is not living. I'll be damned if this thing will trap me. I won't let it come to that. I won't. I'll take care of it before then."

Mom was crying on the couch. She got up and went into the bathroom and returned, eyes puffy and red. "Enough for today," she said. "Okay? Enough."

Pa shook his head. He pulled Kai close to his chest, buried his head in his hair, kissed him, and whispered, "I'll take care of it before then."

16. The Fight

And then Mom found the cure.

Italian researchers were testing a drug on ALS patients that was made by Insmed, and according to Mom's Web search, results were promising. A cure, we all thought. Some hope! She called Pa's doctor, but he said he'd never heard of it. "Shouldn't you know?" Mom asked. "Isn't that your job to at least know what's going on with ALS even if it isn't your trial?" He said he'd get back to her.

We didn't have that sort of time. So Mom continued to investigate, Web page upon Web page. She asked questions on ALS forums. Emailed pharmaceutical companies. Finally a response came from Pa's doctor—information that mirrored Mom's research. The drug hadn't been approved by the FDA, so there was no chance of getting it in the U.S., even on a trial basis for my dad. There was also a legal clash that halted its distribution to patients even if the FDA were to allow it.

"But he's terminal," she argued on the phone. "What's it going to do, kill him? He'd be thankful." The doctor apologized and hung up.

We realized that patients like Pa with terminal orphan diseases (ones that affect less than 200,000 people nationwide and, therefore, aren't highly profitable for pharmaceutical companies) are left to die without much direction or care. After a while the hospital never checked in, called, or offered Mom any help on how to clear an airway when my dad began choking. She had to do all the work, hoping she didn't mess up. She did call upon the ALS Association from time to time because unlike the hospitals, the association was filled with sympathetic individuals who supplied Mom with a variety of resources and equipment, donated from those who "no longer needed it." Lisa, Pa's case manager from the association, would visit the house to assess what Mom needed. They would eventually supply the BiPAP machine, a wheelchair, and laptop for Pa to use. If not for them, Mom would have been left to her own devices, using her own creativity and intuition on how best to keep her husband alive.

And unlike cancer, where there is at least a fight ahead, terminal, incurable diseases are a resignation, a white flag tossed before the game even begins. But even though the doctor said this drug was a dead end, Mom's discovery offered us all something we hadn't had before: a fight. And fight we did.

From: mikehemery@gmail.com
Subject: Iplex.

To: -------@insmed.com, -------@tercica.com

Good morning,

My name is Michael Hemery and my father was diagnosed with ALS this August. He is 60. It is my understanding that there is no cure for ALS, but research shows that Iplex is helping patients in Italy, but due to a lawsuit here in the States, the drug is unavailable.

I am writing a simple request. My father has been a blue collar worker his entire life. Used his hands. He needs to move to be. To exist. He is dying. Knowing there is something out there that could help him, but is locked up in a legal battle, devastates me. To know someone, somewhere is more concerned about money than my father and the other thousands of people who are dying from this disease is unthinkable.

We're desperate. I don't know what to do without him. And I'm begging for this to stop. I'm begging for you, when you wake up in the morning, stretch, brush your teeth, to think what you could do to help my father. Because he struggles to brush his teeth now. Because he limps to my house to see my son. I need my son to know his grandfather. Because I'd hope that when the day comes for you, someone shows you the same mercy. Someone says, yes, life is more important than this house, this car, this lifestyle I live. To know that a man who worked his whole life for others can live a little longer...well...it seems that is the most important thing. Life is the most important thing.

Thank you. I appreciate your honest consideration of this request. I'm scared as hell that this clock is ticking for my dad...and if he can only have a fighting chance. Well, that's all I ask.

Thank you,
Michael Hemery

The family all wrote similar letters to our state representatives, the President, and local media outlets to draw attention to the fight. Friends and colleagues mailed hundreds of letters and fired off email after email on our behalf. My friend Ryan called and said to check my mailbox. He'd left forty-three letters from his family and friends with postage, ready to be mailed. He told me it was my birthday gift that year. A friend of a friend had a contact in Italy. She did legwork for us by contacting the scientists involved in the study. She found out about an upcoming conference on Iplex and ALS and entrenched herself in the battle.

Although my dad continued to decline, we carried on like it wouldn't always be this way because now, for the first time, we understood and could actually see the hope.

Time passed.

The lawsuit cleared.

And the government decided to allow Iplex into the country as long as these terminal patients had a prescription from their doctors. They heard our cry.

Mom called Pa's doctor the day the ban was lifted. We were one signature on a square little slip of paper away from recovery. We all had faith that this version of my dad, clinging to a walker to move ten, eight steps, would eventually be a memory. Muscle would grow over his thinning calves, filling in the gaps.

"The fucker said no." Mom fell onto the couch. "Just like that, he said no. Said he didn't feel it was safe. He's goddamn dying before our eyes and he said it wouldn't be safe. Wouldn't sign the prescription." Her body shook as she cried.

Pa shook his head. "Stop," he said. "You don't know if it will even work."

I said, "I bet we can find someone. Some doctor will sign the prescription. There are doctors that will sign all sorts of prescriptions for people." Mom shook her head.

"That's not the point. It's that they won't even help. They just say 'no' without any kind of other solution. Without any kind of hope. Just 'no' like they don't even care."

"They don't," Pa said. "It's a job. They see dozens of people like me. Nothing new. Nothing real. They get paid to do what they do. Or don't do."

The room was silent. Stacie rubbed Mom's back. Pa looked out the window. "We'll find someone," I said. "Someone will sign it."

But no one would. The few doctors we contacted said they couldn't put their professional careers at stake. Each said that only Pa's doctor could make that call. They each repeated the words *malpractice* and *law-suit*.

We ran out of contacts. For some time I felt like we missed out. Like our chance was there. Pa's life could have been saved, but no one would take a risk. The fight had been knocked out of us.

And then a few weeks later I received an email from my friend in Italy.

> Michael,
>
> I spoke with the doctor who was spearheading the Iplex study here in Italy. He just finished presenting his findings at a conference. I'm so sorry, but he said there was no evidence that the drug helped any of the patients. The positive results that were being posted were simply rumors. The U.S. might still run a trial, but it sounds like it's not going to work. I'm so sorry.

And then the hope had been knocked out of us, too.

17. Slow Descent

Blimps are just begging to be chased. Lumbering in the sky, cruising at a paltry thirty-five miles per hour, my dad and I pursued a blimp for miles when I was eight. We first spotted the hulking beast on the drive home from the lake, surfboards chattering on the roof of the truck. On the drives back and forth to the lake, I'd pretend the two windsurfer masts that peeked over the roof of the cab were gun turrets that lit up when I pressed one of the plastic knockouts on the console where the radio should have been. My dad would make a siren sound, calling out targets—the iron ore factory, McDonald's, the old man who was taking too long to cross the street. I'd press into the console and then join my dad in making explosion sounds, flailing my hands in the air, mimicking the impending explosion. We'd laugh and drive forward, searching for our next mark.

When he called out the blimp at "about eleven o'clock in the sky," I checked my watch to see the direction. I had to squint against the mid-afternoon sun to see the shadow lingering in the sky. We'd shot down all kinds of air-born vehicles—jets, 747s, and even once a helicopter. But the blimp was different. Even after he told me to take aim, I didn't poise my finger ready for an attack. Instead, I shifted forward on the truck bench to get a better view of the blimp.

It didn't even look like it was moving, but instead it just floated like an abstraction, a concept, an unanswered proposal. My dad asked what I was waiting for. I told him a better shot. I said the angle was all wrong. I flicked up my thumb, calculating an imaginary trajectory. I glanced over the tip of my thumb to watch the blimp just exist. I told Pa how I wished all things could be blimp-like. I said I wanted to toss my beach towel in the air, let it remain suspended, never coming down. It would stay afloat so I could walk all around it, crawl underneath to see how its folds looked when frozen in the air. I said I wanted to slow everything down, my towel a magic carpet, suspended indefinitely until I commanded it to fall. Until I shot it down.

My dad turned the steering wheel slightly, the truck crossing the center line a bit. "That's your shot," he said. "Take it." Mom yelled at him for driving carelessly. Said he'd get us all killed. So I pressed the button. I pushed hard, held my finger on the button until the red in my thumbnail turned white. Dad and I made our explosion sounds, and he eased the truck back into our lane.

But unlike our other fatalities, the blimp remained. It didn't disappear like a plane, quickly moving beyond the horizon. It remained frozen. Dad said it must have armor.

So he pressed some buttons near the steering wheel, saying he was reloading the cannons, but this time with death rays, gamma shots, and even a mega bomb. He nodded. I nodded. He told me to take aim. Thumb on the plastic knockout. I waited. Eyed it up. Pressed.

Pa made the explosion sounds, but I just watched, on the edge of the truck seat. The blimp was still some distance away.

"I think it worked that time," Pa said.

I continued to stare.

"What's wrong?" Mom asked.

I pointed at the blimp, which suddenly plunged from its course, dropping from the sky. "I think it worked, too."

Pa explained coincidence—how it wasn't possible. He insisted they were just windsurfer masts on the top of a truck. But he continued to watch with me, looking up from the road as the monster careened to the ground.

We hunted her for miles, and as we neared our home, her terminus became more clear—she was aiming for the small airport just on the outskirts of our neighborhood.

When we pulled in our driveway, Pa parked the truck, and we told Mom we loved her, running hand in hand to the airport. The blimp was on the ground by the time we arrived; three men circled the cockpit prodding, examining. As we approached they nodded.

"Quite a sight to see something this big falling from the sky," Pa said to the man wearing the captain hat.

"Lost power in one of the engines," the man said. "So we made an emergency landing here."

"Did we shoot…" I started to ask Pa, but he squeezed my hand tightly, so I stopped talking.

"We don't get blimps here often," Pa said.

"Imagine not," the man said. "And even if you did, you might not know it because they run so quiet." We could always hear the planes approaching.

Soon a crowd of people gathered around the blimp—men and their sons with lots of questions. A few took their pictures next to the downed elephant.

After nearly an hour, Pa said we needed to get home to clean our surfing gear, take showers, and eat dinner. We thanked the men for their time.

After my shower and dinner I rushed to the front window, hoping to see the blimp's ascent.

An hour later Pa kneeled next to me by the window.

"We didn't make it fall, did we?" I asked.

He shook his head.

"Then how come it broke? I pushed the button for the pretend missile. It didn't become real, did it?"

"No," Pa said, crouching next to me, putting his arm around my shoulders, "sometimes things just break, and it's no one's fault."

18. Transitional Paths

For much of the summer I found immense pleasure in watching my dad mow his lawn. He resembled some sort of cyborg in the command seat of the zero-turn mower. As Joe the salesman promised, the slightest pressure on the steering bars could move the mower. "A fingertip," Joe said, "is all it takes." Pa sprayed poison anywhere he used to trim with the weed whacker, scorching the grass brown, so he didn't have to get off the mower. Mom would still cut a stripe outside the fence and clean up the ditch with the "push" mower, but Pa killed most everything he couldn't tend to personally.

Sitting on my deck, I watched the old man tear across his backyard, completing the job that used to take an hour in less than twenty minutes. For a second I almost convinced myself the disease had made him more powerful. Now, just by twitching his pointer finger, he could almost float across his lawn. Like a god.

Before the mower's arrival I had the gate between our two properties widened so the mower could pass through. I saw no reason why I shouldn't benefit from the speed of the new machine. The new opening cut through my parents' garden, so Pa said, "We'll need to build some sort of transitional path between the two yards using those huge rocks you pulled out of your pond. Otherwise the mower will end up trashing the loose dirt in the garden."

I began the project one afternoon while my parents were away. I hauled two to three rocks at a time in the wheelbarrow to the back of the yard, until I had a nice stack of stone next to the fence. Using a shovel, I dug estimates for each rock and then tapped them into place. A Byzantine mosaic it was not. Several of the stones stuck out at odd heights, but I took some excess mud and tried to build up the gaps into a sloppy seam.

"That's not going to work," Pa said when he returned home and walked into the backyard with his cane that converted into a seat.

I'd been working on the project for much of the afternoon and was exhausted. The idea of restarting was daunting.

"You'll have to make it all even and packed tight, or the mower will push the rocks out of place." Pa lowered himself onto his stool next to the walkway.

"Does it matter?" I asked. "I mean, it's in the back of the yard. No one is going to see it."

Pa shook his head. "That one," he said, pointing to the largest rock in the path.

I pointed to the one I thought he was talking about.

"No," he said, leaning over and picking up a piece of mulch. He underhand tossed it at a stone, the mulch settling on the muddy rock. "That one. Start with that one." I shook my head and wedged the shovel underneath this stone and rocked it out of place. "Now break up that dirt where the stone was, take some of it out, and leave the rest all chopped up so there is a good surface for the stone. Then it won't shift."

"Do we have to do this to all of the stones?" I asked. The path *was* a mess, like tumors growing out of the ground.

"If we're going to do it right," he said. I began breaking up the dirt with the shovel. It was hard and wouldn't crumble easily. The one-by-two space took too long. Too much effort. I rested my elbow on the shovel's handle when the space was clear, sweat beading at my hairline.

"You have like a dozen more," Pa said.

"I know," I replied.

Resting the shovel on the fence, I shoved the rock into place. It was still too high.

"You need to take out more dirt," Pa said.

I popped the stone out of place with the shovel, flipped it over, and began to shovel out more dirt, which then required the remaining dirt to be broken into pieces. I shoved the rock back into place. "More," Pa said.

Stone out. Dirt out. Break into pieces. Stone. "More."

"Fuck," I said. "Seriously, fucking shit, this is going to take all goddamn night. It's fine. It's fine. Who the fuck cares if it's perfect?" I lifted up my shirt to wipe away the sweat.

Pa looked at the path. I looked at the path, its mismatched stones protruding out at various heights. "But it needs to be level so the mower can clear the stones." His voice was small.

I counted the stones. More than a dozen. "It needs to be right," he said.

"It's fine. It's good enough. And I'm not you. I hate this shit. I've always hated this shit. You always have to make this stuff perfect, but you like doing it. I don't. I fucking hate it. I don't care if it's not entirely flat. I just don't care. And I don't want to waste any more of the day doing this just because you need it to be absolutely perfect." I'd forgotten to breathe.

Pa paused for a moment, then said, "You know I'd do it if I could." He used the handle of his chair to adjust his position. He looked up at me. "I know you hate this kind of work. I'd do it for you in a heartbeat. If I could get my body to move or work or anything, I'd lift every stone for you."

"I'm sorry," I said. "I didn't mean it. I know you would."

"Every goddamn stone." He adjusted again. He was beginning to lose more muscle in his core, which caused his body to lurch forward. Without a back on the chair, it was difficult for him to stay upright.

The sun was headed the other way. The late afternoon light sat on the trees' leaves, beginning its slow slide downward. The air was cooler now. I wasn't sweating anymore.

"I'd do it all for you. That's how it's supposed to be. This shouldn't be your problem. None of it should. Make sure Mom learns to use that mower because you shouldn't have to take care of these two yards. You have a family now, and this just isn't how it's supposed to be. I've always taken care of this stuff. I like to. I *liked* to."

I wanted to hold him, to pick him up and hold him, but I knew his body was starting to crush itself. Without muscle, it hurt when he was squeezed too hard. So instead, I picked up the shovel. Removed the stone. Removed the dirt. Crushed what was left. And replaced the stone. It still wasn't right. So I did it again. And again. Until it was perfect.

Pa nodded.

"Why don't you go in? It's hard to sit here, I know."

Pa nodded again. Said he loved me. Hoisted himself out of his chair, collapsed it into a cane.

"You need help?"

He shook his head and slowly worked his way back to the house, taking the long way to avoid the exposed tree roots that he could no longer raise his legs over.

I toiled on, removing the dozen or so stones from the path a dozen or so times until each sat perfectly in line with the other. A perfect path, a transition, from his yard to mine. I hopped on each stone to make sure it didn't rock or give under my weight. Using some of the remaining dirt that I'd piled next to the path, I filled in the gaps like grout, then brushed off each stone.

"I'm impressed," he said. Somehow, hours later, I didn't hear him come back out and shuffle next to me. "Seriously, that's beautiful. I don't think I could have done a better job." He stood, leaning on his cane. His time inside must have refreshed him because he spoke stronger than before. He raised his free hand and placed it on my shoulder. "Maybe there is some hope for you after all." He smiled.

The sun was nearly gone. The light tinted the path a soft, orange tone.

"Should I take some pictures and send them to *Better Homes and Gardens*?" I asked.

I joked about ALS, how at least the disease allowed us to get the zero turn and cut down our yard work time. He repeated that I needed to show Mom how to use it. "I never want you to have two houses to take care of." I smiled and said the only reason I worked so hard on the path was so that he'd be inclined to mow my lawn while I was at work. Which he did. Nearly every week. While I was at work, the old man rode the mower over the path into my yard and took care of me the best his body would still allow.

Everything was coated with death. It lingered on the piano, tucked itself into the cracks in the wall. I needed to go home under the guise of tending to Kai, but in reality I just needed to get out. I kissed Pa on the head and said goodbye. His hair still smelled like him: alive. I promised I'd be back with Kai and Stacie. To say goodbye.

I pulled a bagel from the bag in the kitchen. "I should eat," I said to Mom, who followed into the other room. "You should eat. Even if you don't want to. This is going to be a long day."

She leaned into my chest and sobbed. I kissed the top of her head. "It was never supposed to be like this," she said. "Never."

"Now what?" I asked.

"I don't know."

"You called the doctor?"

She nodded her head, wiping her face dry. Pa's mask hissed from the living room. I stepped back. His eyes were closed—the room still lit by a single light.

"Maybe the doctor will say no," she said. "They don't just let people die like that, I don't think."

"It's probably just like removing life support. They do. So now what?"

"I guess we wait and see what they say. Pa's plan is to have enough morphine to pass out. Then we remove the mask while he sleeps."

He took morphine for the first time two days prior when the pain was too much. It was the first time he took it, even though Lisa told him there was nothing wrong with feeling relief and he should consider an occasional dose. But he never took it. He said he never wanted to miss a thing, even in the state he was in. When he did eventually take a small dose, it wiped him out. He passed out for nearly a day. Mom kept checking to make sure he was still alive, but he'd just entered a deep, restful sleep, void of the usual pain his body offered.

I don't believe he took it that day because of the pain—I think he wanted to take a test run of the process he'd been concocting in his brain to see if it would do the job when he needed it to.

"He wants this?" I asked.

"More than anything," Mom answered.

"I don't know how I'm going to do this without him."

Mom wiped her face onto her sleeve. "None of us do," she said. "Go."

"Are you okay?"

"No. Go."

"I'll get those two and be right back."

"Come back later," she said. "It's not going to be right now. It'll take time for approvals and signatures and okays to let him die."

She looked into my eyes and repeated it. "To let him die." Her eyes were red and at that moment I heard that word for the first time for what it really meant. Short. Concise. To the point. *Die.*

"Go." She helped me with my sweatshirt. Hugged me. And said she'd be fine. I went back into the living room and kissed Pa's head again. His eyes were still closed, but he nodded his head ever so slightly. His skull even seemed frail. Like the bone could break under the weight of my lips. He opened his eyes, mouthed I love you through his mask, and closed his eyes again, waving ever so slightly with his hand—the only movement he had left.

19. Father's Day

Mom bought him a weeding stool. We visited three different stores when Mom asked, "Is this crazy?"

"To buy your soon-to-be crippled husband a weeding stool for Father's Day?" I asked.

"Stop saying it like that," she said, laughing. "No seriously—he just keeps trying to do everything—to keep doing everything he used to. The other day I found him on his knees crawling to weed the backyard. That's insane."

"Not nearly as insane as buying him a weeding stool instead of just doing the weeding for him." We both laughed, but knew this was the perfect gift for him. He didn't want anyone else to do it. He wanted to yank every piece of clover out of his garden beds himself—otherwise he'd just be irritated with our shoddy work.

Before the zero turn was delivered I mowed his yard for him once. On my way out he said, "They are only giving me two years to live, but I guarantee you'll have less if you screw up my yard." So Mom and I tested a dozen gardening stools, sitting our butts on them, trying to imagine what his course around the yard would be like without working legs. We finally found one with wheels so he could push or pull himself around the yard without getting up.

"I'm worried about the wheels," Mom said. "They might not go over the dirt."

"Maybe you could just push him—like give him a good shove." She hit me on the head.

Pa laughed so hard on Father's Day when he opened the stool I was worried we were going to lead him to an earlier death. Although he laughed, he must have been anxious to try it out because that afternoon he pushed himself around the back patio to weed the beds. I walked over to their yard when I heard him shouting for Mom. They were both near tears of laughter because one of the wheels was wedged in a crack on the patio, and he didn't have the strength to push himself, nor could he crawl out of the seat. "I told you, Mom. All he needs is a good shove."

I perched on their back step and Mom sat in her lawn chair, while my dad continued to work his way around the beds. "This is quite the scene," he said. "The old man with ALS doing all the work to keep this house in shape while you bastards watch." He laughed so hard he needed to take a break from the weeding.

After a few minutes the phone rang and Mom handed it to my dad. It was the psychologist from the hospital, who checked in a few times to make sure my dad wasn't going to kill himself. She always led with the same question: "Do you ever have thoughts of harming yourself?" And my dad answered every time with, "Every day."

She then asked if people were helping my dad get around and take care of tasks like preparing meals and showering. "You bet," my dad said on the phone. "In fact, my kid and wife just bought me a stool with wheels so I can weed the garden beds." He said the psychologist asked if he was kidding. "Nope." He held the phone to the wheels and moved back and forth, the plastic snapping against the cement. "Can you hear that? Wheels."

She then asked if someone was helping his wife during this time. "Yeah, me. I'm doing the laundry, weeding, mowing the lawn."

After he hung up and recounted the story I said, "Now wait a minute, who put that stool together? Your hands weren't going to screw those screws in. Where is my thanks? I'm happy to help—not with the actual weeding, of course—but I can put stools together."

"Whoah, whoah, whoah," Pa said, "yeah, let's not get crazy—weeding? That would just be crazy."

After more laughter, I went home for lunch, but returned later that evening to check on the status of the yard. My dad was still outside, but now in the farthest end of the yard, resting his arm on the stool. He was kneeling in the dirt with one hand on the stool for balance.

"Why aren't you rolling around on that thing?" I asked.

"Doesn't move well in the grass," he said. "But don't tell your mother. It was sweet of her to try." I nodded. He bit his lip and surveyed the garden beds. "This takes forever now. Used to knock this out in an afternoon." The plastic bucket by his side was only half full of weeds.

"Move over," I said. I started to yank weeds and throw them in the bucket.

"I don't want you to do this," Pa said.

"Neither do I." I smiled.

"Seriously, go home. I was just kidding before—I can do this."

"By the time you're done with the yard new weeds will grow where you started."

"You suck."

"Watch it or I'll stick you on that stool and shove you down the driveway."

"I really don't want your help," he said, returning to weeding.

"I know," I said. "I just want to put on a good show in case the hospital sends someone over to check on patient abuse."

We worked that way well into the evening, until the bucket was brimming with weeds and the yard looked as tidy and perfect as ever.

20. Passing Moment

To celebrate Mom's birthday, the family, including my paternal grandmother, ate dinner at Quince, an upscale restaurant near our homes. My grandma never adjusted to the news. Though, to be fair, none of us really did. But she never learned to even exist within the world where her son was dying. Pa held back the truths of the disease in the beginning—never using the words *paralyzed* or *death*. But when she mentioned ALS to someone she befriended at the nursing home where my grandpa lived, that woman gave her all the grim details. It was that day she was no longer able to work her way into my parents' lives without staring at my dad with *those* eyes—like death was imminent after every breath. She was also unable to talk about *it* with him. This day was no different; she never whispered a word of the future.

For us, each celebration became painful because we all worried this would be the last one: the last birthday he'd watch Mom blow out the candles or the last Christmas he'd tear open a gift (or watch someone tear open a gift when his hands gave out). I became obsessed with taking photos of every moment. I took so many pictures of him with Kai, smiling. I believed I was taking them for Kai, so he'd remember what it looked like when he sat on Papa's lap, shouting "There's a car" at the passing vehicles outside Pa's front window. But maybe I knew they were for me, too. So I'd remember what his smile looked like.

During dinner Pa fidgeted on the wooden chair, his spine and bones no longer encased in much muscle, but exposed to whatever surface they came into contact with. After the main course Grandma said she'd buy dessert, if we wanted, but I recommended we go for a walk to the ice cream shop across from the restaurant. "Can you make it?" I asked Pa. He nodded.

The late-afternoon sun was exceptional that evening. Like the day Kai was born, a warm light made extended shadows on the ground and tinted the grass a rich green hue. I've been aware of light as long as I've been a photographer, preferring the pronounced shadows of fall over the brightness of spring. I'd tried to shoot like a contemporary Caravaggio painting. That afternoon the shadows even buried themselves in the bricks, each an object my dad could potentially trip over. But he made it and slumped in a more rounded mesh chair that contoured to the curve of his spine. And he smiled, his face directly pointing at the sun in a way that actually washed away the shadows of his sunken eyes. I reached for the camera in my pocket, but realized I'd left it at home. That smile is one I would have wanted to keep.

Kai giggled in his stroller, Mom pushing him up and down the path, bouncing on each brick. We ate ice cream. Some dribbled down Stacie's chin, and Pa laughed—not the struggled gasps he'd been offering, but a real laugh, from somewhere much stronger. There was no one else in the courtyard that evening, other than a few sparrows that played on a horse buggy that rested in the grass.

"It's really good," Pa said, finishing the rest of his cone. He leaned back and closed his eyes against the sun. We talked about ice cream flavors and the upcoming football season. Grandma said the Browns weren't going to be any good this year. I said they never were, but we'd watch anyhow because what else was there to look forward to on Sunday afternoons? Although the quilting store had been closed for hours, Stacie peeked in the windows with Mom, pointing to fabrics she wanted to use in our friend's baby blanket. Pa called out different planes overhead to Kai, who listened with wonder at Pa's explanation of the differences between propeller planes and jets. Not even a year old, but he was already enamored with cars and planes, or whatever else my dad said. And when the trains, whose tracks were cut a few dozen feet from where we were sitting, tore by with all their horns and bells and energy, we stopped. Because we had to. Stacie covered Kai's ears. The rest of us paused mid speech, and we watched one another. We couldn't see the trains behind the buildings; we could only hear their momentum. And as soon as they passed, so did our suspended animation. We went back to banter about traffic patterns, lawn fertilizers, and sewing machines.

That entire evening we spoke like *it* wasn't there. I think we'd all forgotten. Because of the light. Sounds. Each other. And in that moment, I realized that's all we ever have: that moment. That one single breath of perfection when there was no rot in any of us, only a completely perfect slice of time. Yeats' damn rose, but we touched it, smelled it, plucked it as our own. As it was happening, I think we all knew that those minutes in that courtyard, the trickle of water from the nearby waterfall and the rustle of laughter in our throats, was everything. Because, after all, that's all we actually have are those moments—before the bills beg to be paid, before the emergency rush to the hospital, before the glass accidentally falls from the cupboard onto the ground, erupting into splinters of clear sand and fragments of frustration. That moment. Those minutes. That day. It's all we have. It's all we've ever had. I didn't think about how hard it would be for him to stand up out of the mesh chair in fifteen minutes or the lifespan of the sparrows who pecked at the seeds beneath the carriage. Instead I lived, possibly for the first time, in that moment, experiencing the closest thing I'd ever witnessed to pure love.

The forgotten camera meant no images of that perfect light. But maybe that is best, because that day is forever documented within us all, a moment when even the deepest shadows were filled with light.

When I returned home from my parents' house Kai was waiting for me in the living room.

"Wus wrong?" he asked. "Crying? Wus wrong? Hugs?"

He trotted across the room and offered his hands, outstretched. I fell to my knees and hugged him as tightly as I could, but no matter how hard I tried, he was never close enough.

21. The Business of Death

The number of walks through the backyard declined. After finishing the path for the lawnmower, my dad helped me build new doors for my shed—the others rotted through. He made it into my yard and would breathe out directions—what to cut and how.

Since I didn't know the first thing about constructing anything, I became an extension of his dead arms. Whenever I tried to go rogue, I slipped up. "You have to measure the length of the two-by-fours exactly, otherwise nothing will fit!" I nodded. I knew he was right. So I remeasured the two-by-fours and followed his directions precisely. After the doors were constructed and trimmed, he walked me through the process of hanging them. They fit tighter than the old ones. They fit perfectly—there was no longer even a dime-size gap for the pesky mice to slip through. "You paint them," he said on the last day. "I'm going home."

We worked this way for a month. He called me over to replace the water filter under the sink and explained how to remove the battery from the lawnmower in the winter. He described how the filter slipped into the track of his furnace. He reminded me the driveway markers went in after the very last mow of the season, before the ground froze, and that the mower should be at the lowest height for that last mow. And when mice made their way into our siding, he came over, smacking his cane into the side of the house, trying to pinpoint their exact position. "I wish I could help you more, kiddo," he said that night. It was getting dark. The mice were louder now, even ignoring my kicks on the side of the house. "But I just can't move my body anymore. But you know what to do—traps. Dozens of traps, until you get every last one of them." I made a face. I detested the way the traps caught the mice in the back of the necks, the trails of blood that came from their mouths, the flopping of their dying bodies. "It's you or them. You can't live together." The noise in the siding grew bolder. I gave the siding a final kick, but failed to hush the critters. The two of us sat outside until the moonlight provided the only light, talking about the tree house we built together when I was six, listening to scampering of tiny feet against aluminum.

In the early fall he made me grease and change the oil in the snow blower. The process was awkward—I had no idea how to connect the grease gun to the machine. But he was patient. When I failed, he made me do it again. I didn't correctly connect the hose to the fitting and grease sprayed across the garage. He made me do it again until the machine was greased. "You need to know how to do this stuff," he said. "You'll have to do it." He wasn't asking for help. He could probably still manage to squeeze the gun with two hands. No, he was training me, passing along the basic skills so his home would exist beyond his own breaths. So Mom would be taken care of. "Start it up," he said. I pulled the cable, but the engine bogged. I looked at him. "Again," he instructed. This time the engine stuttered, but gained momentum and eventually caught its stride and ran. *It ran.* Even though the floor was covered in brown grease, he nodded when I was done, and said, "That's my boy." He smiled and seemed content.

He was sharing all he knew. I wondered what I would show my son if I knew the end was near. If I had the time to decide what was really important in life. In those days when my dad could still move, he transferred a lifetime of knowledge about machines and the home, the basics that keep life moving forward with fewer complications.

He still mowed the lawn for the remainder of that season. The mower offered speed and movement. I loved watching him cut across the yards effortlessly, like a superhero—the machine guided by the flick of his fingers. The last time he walked through the yards to our house was for the first pregame of the Browns season. He used his walker, taking breaks throughout the yard. I helped him up the stairs of the deck, and he slumped onto the couch. He didn't have the strength to lower himself anymore. It was a plop. Kai, who was turning one, played at his feet, and pulled himself up on the couch. My dad lowered his head to Kai and my son gently pressed his head into my dad's. And there the two of them rested, for several seconds, as if they were saying *I love you.* As if my dad was transferring all he knew or felt to Kai, the only way he could. Kai laughed—he always did when my dad was around—and eased himself back onto the floor to play with the toys scattered about.

"It's getting harder," my dad said.

I nodded. "You want a beer?" I asked.

"I can't anymore. It's hard to swallow for some reason. Too thick."

"I'm so sorry."

"Nah, it's not like that. It's just hard to move. Everything is pain now. Frustrating just to walk across the stupid yard." He paused. "I can still drink wine though. At least this stupid disease hasn't taken that."

"You want some?" I asked, making a move for the kitchen.

"Not today," he said. "I just want to sit here in the sun today." Light streamed in my front bay window and made long lines on his skin.

Kai picked up an orange ball and tossed it at my dad. Pa smiled and pushed it off the couch with the back of his hand, Kai quickly scampering after it. Pa looked tired. His one eye was smaller than the other. The skin on his thinning face hung off his cheekbones more.

"Mom says she has *the* pill," Pa finally said.

"*The* pill?" I asked. "Like, the one to off you?"

"That's what I asked." He laughed. "No, she thinks she has some new vitamin that will work."

"Worth a shot."

"If there was an answer, they'd have found it. If this were contagious, they would have fixed it." I nodded. "But it's not. Not enough people have it, so they don't waste much money on figuring it out, I guess. I never did anything wrong, you know." I said I knew that. "They can fix people who get all these diseases from messing around, but they can't fix this."

The ball hit him in the face. He gave Kai a stern look and then immediately laughed. Kai giggled and clapped his hands together. "Ball," Kai said. "Ball."

"That kid of yours is so smart. Watch him. He's going to be too smart. Smarter than me and you. Be careful when he gets older." The subtext was always a reminder—he wouldn't be there when Kai was older. We had to acknowledge that in our exchanges. I understood what was happening cognitively, but I squelched the emotions, like some kind of dam. I could discuss his death, the future, as a matter of business, like changing tires on a car, because I could block off the feeling. I couldn't cry in front of him anymore. He didn't need that. And like a dam, I allowed those feelings later, when he left, when Stacie could hold my shuddering body in bed. So we talked about the business—watching my son's smarts, greasing snow blowers, and measuring two-by-fours.

"And he has a great laugh," Pa said. "He's funny because he's smart. Those two usually go hand in hand. But I love that laugh. Kids' laughter is the best." He began telling me a story about the days when he worked at Gowe Printing—a filthy, horrible job that he hated. He'd slave for the company, working dozens of hours of overtime, only to worry and stress. He said those were the worst years of his life. "But I loved one part of that place," he said. "At lunch I'd go outside just to get out and I'd hear these kids at some playground nearby. I could never see them, only hear them. I swore I'd get out of there someday—go someplace where I could hear kids laughing while I worked. It just makes everything better. Maybe that's why I started working as a janitor for the schools—because when a kid laughs you believe everything will work out in the end."

The football game was only a distraction. We never watched seriously, because we knew the Browns would ultimately lose. So we talked about the mold in my windows—if I needed new ones soon. All the while, he played catch with my son, for nearly an hour, until my dad said he should mosey home. "Not that I can get home any other way than moseying," he said with a laugh. He called Kai to the couch one more time, pressing his forehead into Kai's. My dad raised his head, cradled my son's head in his hands and kissed it. Kai scooted across the couch and threw his hands around my dad's leg, hugging him. I forced the tears to remain still.

After Kai let go, I helped Pa up from the couch, walked with him onto the deck, and helped him down the stairs.

"You want me to walk with you?" I asked.

"Nah," he said. "I got this."

So, I went back inside and watched him "mosey" his way across my backyard. He'd stop every few steps to breathe, looking up at the sky, a brighter blue than it had been in some time. Although I didn't know while I watched out the kitchen window, this was the last time he'd ever walk home from my house.

22. Achieving Normal

I'd only ambled through the yard to borrow some eggs from my folks on an abnormally frigid September afternoon when I discovered them huddled on milk crates, wearing thick down winter jackets and drinking wine on their back patio.

"What the hell are you two doing?" I asked.

Mom laughed. Her eyes were red—she'd been crying. But now she laughed, her arm hooked around my dad's.

"Have you two lost it? Because it seems like you've lost it."

Pa raised the glass to his lips and smiled. He had to switch glasses, because he could no longer sip from the thin-stemmed variety, so he now sloshed his wine in an old, orange plastic cup chewed about the rim.

"What?" he asked. "You took away all our furniture, so where else were we going to sit?" I'd stored all their lawn furniture for the winter in my shed—a task my dad used to be in charge of.

"It's cold. Go inside."

"The sun feels good," Mom said. Despite her eyes, she smiled a sincere smile. The process had been wearing on her—the daily taking its toll. Because of the need for healthcare, she was forced to return to work at the elementary school down the street from her house, which meant my dad was alone during the day. Still on maternity leave, Stacie would walk through the backyard with Kai nearly every afternoon, but Mom said she worried about my dad alone in the house. He was still able to navigate, albeit slowly, to the kitchen to gather his lunch and could make his way to the bathroom. But it was becoming more problematic. Mom was short on the phone now when I called. There was business to attend to when she came home. Aside from preparing dinner and tending to all the house chores, she had to continue researching medical trials that might offer some hope.

But this afternoon, those worries seemed somewhere else. Maybe the buzz from the wine set her smile right, but it was fueled by some greater peace, surely. The two of them would frequently eat on the patios of various restaurants well past the outdoor-eating season. They'd been known to enjoy breakfast at local bagel shops while snow dotted their food. They always were disposed to the bitter temperatures, so outdoor dining in the winter seemed utterly normal. And maybe that's why Mom smiled that afternoon—because it seemed normal. A glass of Cabernet on the patio, while sitting on milk crates—perhaps that was the furthest point from that "thing" that lingered inside the house.

"You're not right," I said. "Neither of you. You're going to get sick out here."

"Hope I don't catch something that will kill me," Pa said, laughing. Mom smacked him on the shoulder and chuckled.

"You see this?" Pa pointed to the stroller near him. "Your mother suggested I use this to move around now." He pretended to stab himself in the eye with the handle of the stroller. "Kill me now."

"Don't tempt me," Mom said. "You're a real pain in the ass with this fumbling around you're doing." They laughed their cheeks red.

"Well, I'm getting my eggs and going home," I said. "There is nothing normal about you two."

Mom nestled her arm further into my dad's. She giggled and took another sip of her wine, resting her head on his shoulder.

23. The Shoulders of a God

One of my first childhood memories is the taste of his hair. How it would absorb the sun on our walks down the railroad, no real destination—his body moving over railroad ties in an extended gait. Me, balanced on his shoulders, legs dangling down his chest—I'd fall asleep up there, his jet-black hair hot against my cheek, as I'd be lulled to rest. They'd joke about how I could fall asleep on these long walks, my dad shouldering my weight, literally, for miles. "You'd even drool sometimes," Mom said. "But he never had the heart to wake you. You always looked too comfortable riding up there, like a king—on the shoulders of a god."

We surely completed some simple tasks—fed Kai, dressed him. But every movement just delayed us from going back. There was a rush to return to my parents' house because any moment we weren't there was one less moment with him.

The sun rose by the time we pulled up to their driveway. Kai rushed in the side door and shouted "Papa!" as he rounded the corner into the living room—just as he did every time we entered their house. He loved my dad—the two connected on a level no one else could understand. They'd watch cars out the front window for hours. Pa pointing. Kai saying, "There'sacar!" I worried about our kiddo, his routines and how he'd deal with the loss of my dad. Tomorrow he'd turn that corner and be struck with an empty seat—my dad's place for most of Kai's life. My old man taught him to crawl. When his legs began failing and he'd be on the floor playing cars with Kai, struggling to get back to his seat, he'd say, "This is how you crawl, kiddo," moving his body to his chair so he could pull himself back into place. But I also knew Kai would adapt. He was still young and didn't quite get it. I worried more about me—how I'd deal with that moment when Kai turned the corner, shouting my dad's name at an empty chair.

The mood was lighter in the sunlight. Too light. Pa smiled more than I'd seen him smile in months. He wore the partial mask and cradled Kai with his working hand. Kai rested his head on Pa's lap and said "love" over and over. "Love," Pa repeated back through the whispers of his mask.

Stacie sat next to Pa's leg, holding him close, and she began crying. He cradled her head the same way. "It's the right thing, kiddo," he said. "I can't go on like this. It's okay. I love you." Stacie gripped his leg and rocked through her tears.

"I just picked out a new book for us," Mom said to me in the kitchen. At night Mom had been reading to him before bed. The previous night they'd just finished *Travels With Charley*. "I was thinking maybe our next one might be *Grapes of Wrath* since it would take us a while. Seemed like a long one. I want more time." She cried into my shoulder again.

She straightened her back and wiped her eyes. "We made the call," she said. The nurse said hospice, who was just assigned to my dad's case a few weeks before, would be contacted. Pa's doctor had to sign off. "But yeah," she said. "The nurse said he'd sign off." Not a matter of if, just when. We cried some more. "They'll give enough morphine to knock him out," Mom explained, "remove the mask, and then wait six minutes."

24. Government Restrictions

"I hate the goddamn government," Pa said, trying to spill gas into the zero-turn mower. I'd just stopped by to check on him—and found him cursing away in the garage.

"Seriously—you want to get rich? Start a store for people like me who have been doing the same thing for the past fifty years. Look at this." He pointed to the nozzle of his new gas can. "The guy at the hardware store said they are only allowed to sell these new cans because people were blowing themselves up or something. How the fuck am I supposed to get this thing open?" The new cans had a pressure point that needed to be in contact with the rim of the tank—you couldn't just open the end and pour anymore. "Seriously—what a great business idea—a store where they sell old stuff, how it used to be done before some idiot sued someone and now they have to put locks and check valves on everything. Can you imagine the money in that? I'd shop at a place that sold the old gas cans right now. I'd drive three hours to go to that store any day of the week over this mess."

I took the can from him, pressing it hard into the tank. The gasoline flowed, albeit with some effort, even for me. There was no way my dad, his hands bricking, could maneuver the spout. He sat on the chair he had set up next to the mower.

"Total bullshit, I tell you," he said. "Same as that thing." He pointed to his Civic hybrid car parked in the garage.

"Oh, right, the 'Cadillac' converter," I said. He smiled.

"There is a tour I could take, you know. In Greenland—they let people kill themselves. All sorts of people from the States are taking it because they say it's illegal for someone to help you."

"You've mentioned it, but c'mon, Pops, this sort of talk is depressing."

"Well, hell yeah it's depressing—this whole fucking mess is depressing. But I just watched a movie on Kevorkian. That guy got it. Good damn movie." Stacie and I bought my parents a subscription to Netflix for Easter. We figured they could at least escape for a bit in a movie a few times a month. We never realized how important those movies would be. My dad never watched a lot of TV—we never had cable. But when he found out he could stream movies on his laptop, he'd sometimes watch four a day because, as he said, "There's not much else to do when your body won't work." But he said it was one of the few pleasures that kept him sane those years.

"Of course he got it," I said. "People should be allowed...they should be able to do whatever they want."

"I'd start up that car right now and do it if I could."

"Would you wait for me to leave, at least," I said. "I don't have a death wish." He smiled again.

"I've looked into how to do it," he said.

I finished filling the tank and placed the can back in its spot at the back of the garage. "I'm sure you have."

"No, seriously, I've looked into all kinds of things." He repeated these suicide stories often.

I could tell Pa wasn't finished with this, so I settled down on the garage step, rested against the door, and let Pa explain all the ways he'd like to commit suicide. After telling me about a variety of ways to end your life, he took a long breath. Talking wore out his core. "It's still just not right. They should let people decide if we want to die. None of them would live with this." I shook my head. "None of them." He breathed hard. "It doesn't matter anyways. I'll figure it out. I won't be a burden on any of you—I'll take care of it on my own."

"I know, Pops," I said. I did know.

I thought about his disease all the time, but I didn't know whom to contact or how to help. I wanted my dad to live. I wondered why extensive research wasn't being conducted every second of every day for such a truly merciless disease. The old man was probably right. About everything—the government, the apathetic attitude toward orphan diseases, even his promise to end it his way. He must have been growing tired—he told me I could go as he straightened out his back.

"If it's okay, I'd like to just sit here for a while," I said.

"I can't talk anymore," my dad said, breathing deeply. "Core is shot."

"I know. We don't have to," I said.

I never imagined sitting in the garage discussing my father's suicide. My favorite memory of that garage was the time he made fishing rods during a downpour. We sat, cozy in the dry of that space, lit by a few hanging lights my dad hung from the rafters. He spun the rods while I played cars near the cracked-open door. He told me to stay out of the rain because I'd catch a cold if I was wet. That space felt safe and holy—like we somehow avoided the lightning and darkness outside. It was the afternoon, but the sky outside that day was darkness. Despite the cracks of thunder I knew I was safe in that space—WMMS, the Cleveland rock station, playing the classics, and my father forging fishing rods from raw materials.

And then again, many years later, I still found solace in that space, in just knowing we shared the garage again for some time, protected from everything on the outside, even if only for a few moments. Because I knew in those moments and in that space we both breathed. Lived. Existed. Because I knew that might be all we had until my dad kept his promise and took care of it.

25. Cleared

The rest of the year ticked away quickly, and my dad's world shrank. There was only one chair in the living room that supported the deterioration. The kind souls at the ALS Association brought over a variety of house chairs, wheelchairs, and pads, but they all presented some kind of nagging pain. There are a "lucky" few who tell their stories of ALS laced with hope (bucket lists and exotic vacations), but the reality for many with this disease is chronic pain, distress, and isolation. Surprisingly, the old suede recliner that sat in the corner of my parents' living room since I was a child was it, the only comfort my dad would find. He'd spend nearly every waking hour in that chair watching Netflix on his ALS Association-provided laptop or the guy across the street mow his yard or wax his car. I took over his yard work for the fall because he was no longer able to pull himself onto the mower. So he'd watch me run lines in the yard. "I'd give anything to be back out there," he told me once when I finished. "Anything to be moving in the world again."

I tried to stop by every day and made up reasons when I had no real agenda. One day I showed my dad new pants I'd purchased for work. He and Mom were eating dinner—all meals were served in the recliner because he couldn't sit upright in the rigid kitchen chairs. I was telling Pa about my students at school, hoping the stories could provide something, anything. He'd just finished eating his last forkful of food when he lurched his body backward, eyes wide open, and began pointing to his chest. He was choking in silence, because his body lacked the muscle strength to heave. "Mom!" I screamed. She was in the kitchen cleaning dishes. "Mom, now, help!"

I stood next to him, but had no idea what to do. The Heimlich would break his fragile bones. So I tapped his back. He gasped as hard as he could. "Mom!" She came rushing in, immediately sliding to her knees next to him and lifting his body from his armpits, stretching out his torso. He let out a moan, and then something emitted a wet click from his throat. The food matter passed. And he breathed again. "Goddammit," Mom said. "Goddammit." She stood up and threw the rag that was slung over her shoulder at the couch. Her fear manifested itself in anger that year. Lots of anger.

"It's okay," Pa whispered, his throat sounding raw. "It's done."

Mom picked up the rag and stomped back into the kitchen. She turned the water back on and returned to the dishes. Her eyes were darker than I'd ever seen—some sort of mix between sadness and rage. Everything they'd heard about—the terrifying symptoms—were starting to manifest themselves. Mom couldn't ignore it anymore, and it broke her somewhere deep inside.

I still stood, frozen, next to my old man. He reached up and took my hand. "It's all bett..." He choked. "Bett..." Again. "Better."

"I know, Pa. Don't talk. It's okay."

"We'll be okay," he struggled out.

"Please stop trying to talk."

"It's done. Don't worry. It's done." He cleared his throat and squeezed my hand. I grew aware of his grip. We all knew that grip wouldn't last another year. But at that moment I knew I had his touch. At that moment he cleared the food from his throat. I was aware that he might not be able to tomorrow. But today he did. Time was something that slipped before and after the present, but it was also something that didn't matter much. What mattered was the still-warm skin of my dying father against my skin.

26. What's New

I still asked him what was new whenever I called. He tolerated the question for months until one day he said, "How much can be new? Mom gets me up, helps me to the chair. I fight to get to the kitchen for lunch by myself and watch movies all damn day because I can't walk. Nothing will ever be new."

"I know. I guess I just want to hear about the movies or whatever you saw out the window."

"It's weird, you know how I can't listen to music anymore," he began. And with that we talked civilly to each other again. It was normal to snap those days. Facing certain death, life became tedious for us all. But he began telling me again how music made him sick to his stomach. "But the movies—thank you for Netflix—I have no idea what I'd do without it. And there are some great movies." He told me about the sailing flicks and the *Bourne* series (his favorite movies of all time). We spoke about what was new, for him.

The next day I asked again, "What's new?"

"I started pole vaulting today," he said.

"What?"

"I knew you wouldn't stop asking, so I figured I'll start giving you answers to keep you happy." The next day it was lifting weights, the next parasailing.

The following day he was out of breath when he answered—he and

Mom had just returned from the pulmonologist downtown. "You tired from the day?" I asked.

"No, because I decided to run behind the car on the way home—figured I could use the exercise." He laughed, but sounded tired. The doctor still insisted Pa make the trip to downtown Cleveland so they could test his breathing levels—data they were using to document the effects of ALS, not information to help him. It was excruciating for him; the angle of the seat in the car made it nearly impossible to take breaths. Mom said he gasped the whole way. Pa said the doctor had a weak handshake. He laughed when he told me that. "Hell, I can squeeze harder than him. Turns out he was a concert pianist. Suppose his hands were important." Mom had lots of questions—how to clear food, how he could cough better and not choke. The doctor didn't have many answers. At all.

"Not a goddamn piece of practical help," Mom said. "They just want to watch him like some sort of lab monkey. They measure everything and say he's getting worse. We know that—don't need a machine to tell me his breathing is getting worse. This was the last time. We're not doing that again. Not for them."

Pa said it was like no one had ever asked the doctors how to cope before. The medical staff didn't have any advice so they recommended the ALS Association. Mom told them they'd already contacted them and they'd been the greatest resource, not the hospital. The doctor said with terminal diseases, they didn't have much to offer. They didn't seem to be in the business of helping those who were untreatable.

That night Mom went online and learned the proper way for Pa to cough. She looked up methods to clear food lodged in his throat as well. Pa said while she was doing that he looked up new ways to kill himself.

Time moved unfairly. That moment, the one I'd learned to respect and appreciate so greatly in the past two years, refused to remain still. I became not only aware, but obsessed with the future—ten minutes from then, the next morning. I felt the minutes, seconds charge forward—by the time I noticed my father's touch, his breaths, his blinks, they were gone. I reminded myself, *I have this moment, I have this moment*, but I didn't. I had nothing, because time refused to linger, but slipped through the air.

Stacie, Mom, Kai and I moved from room to room while we waited for phone calls and further instructions. Pa was light that day—the first hope he'd had in months was death. We still were waiting on a call from the social worker. The doctor approved the removal of the BiPAP, but she still needed to sign off. And she hadn't, yet. It wasn't that she refused, but she just hadn't returned the call.

Aunt Vicki stopped by to print something off on her sister's printer, surely not expecting a home full of people on a work day. I was camped in my parents' office while my dad rested. Kai napped in my parents' bedroom with Stacie. The house was quiet when she came in, but Mom couldn't tell her. She started and stopped but couldn't get it out, so Aunt Vicki came down the hall into the office and I explained everything. The decision. The wait. The social worker.

And then the phone rang. I could only hear Mom's end. "Yes. Yes. I understand." I came down the hall—Pa woke up to listen. He winked at me. Mom stood in the living room, pacing as she spoke. "So hospice will come later? I understand." She set the phone on the end table and sat on the couch.

She looked at Pa; he still wore his breathing mask, so he raised his eyebrows in inquiry. "That was the social worker. She said you're not depressed and that you're making this decision of sound mind."

Pa mouthed, "No shit" through his mask and smiled.

Mom remained composed while she spoke—almost robotic. Aunt Vicki waited in the office, presumably unable to confront any of this. It was a surprise to everyone. We knew it was coming, but no one knew today was the day. "Hospice will be here in a few hours." It was still early afternoon, so I counted the moments I'd have left with him. "The plan is what you said—enough morphine to knock you out, and then they'll remove it." She breathed. "This is what you want? You're sure?"

Pa nodded. He raised his hand to his heart and mouthed through the mask to his wife, "I love you."

27. Christmas Wish

We stumbled into the conversation quite by accident. It was one of those rare times when Pa and I were alone—Stacie, Mom and Kai went shopping for this or that, and he and I somehow moved our conversation to the meaning of life. "You ever wonder about it?" he asked.

"About what?" I lay on the couch, looking at my old man in his chair.

"The whole thing. God. It all."

"All the time; you know that." I was the reason the family stopped going to church. A few college classes on the historical Jesus were enough to crush my faith in magic and miracles, but bolster my admiration for the political revolutionary that was Jesus. After my folks read authors like Crossan and Borg, they agreed that this way was better, and from then on we spent Sundays at home.

"But, I mean, now I have a lot of time, and if there is a God I just want to know how it works. I mean, I can't figure it out. There is always a reason, you know?"

I nodded, fidgeting with the hem of my shirt.

"Like, before you were born, you know how Mom had that miscarriage. I was so mad at God. I'd pray every night and tried to figure it out because there had to be a reason. And then you came, and it all made sense. For me it was like there was probably something wrong with that other kid and when we got you, I mean, look at you, you're perfect. You always have been. So there was a reason and I understood."

"I don't know if it's always that easy, though."

"But it has always made sense. When I quit my job at the printing press, that shit job, I was able to find something else and it was cleaning floors, but it worked itself into that IT job. And it was for a reason." He paused. "I can't see any reason for this. I can't figure out why I have to die."

I couldn't answer, as my throat locked when he said the word "Die." So I grunted and shook my head. Holding back the tears the best I could, choking down the word until I was numb.

"If He picks and chooses," Pa continued, "I keep thinking maybe He'll just take Grandpa. He's sick. He's lived. And maybe this Christmas He'll decide to let me live. A miracle or something. That would be good. Something that just stops it. Wonder if it works like that—if He could just pick."

"It hurts too much to think there is something out there that is cruel enough to let someone like you die or even suffer like you have. I don't buy that. It's probably a lot more random than that. Just nature, chance. An indifferent universe."

"That's a lot harder to take."

I nodded. We sat there for a bit. I couldn't look up—couldn't see his face.

"You know what's odd. For years I've had dreams that I was paralyzed—I'd wake up in a panic, thinking I couldn't move. And now it's so weird, now I have dreams that I'm better. I wake up and think I can just hop out of bed. But when I wake up, I'm smacked with the reality that everything is broken."

I wished I had more to say. I don't think he expected me to respond. Maybe he just needed to say it—to get it out there. So I listened.

"I'd like Him to decide either way by Christmas. I don't want to put Mom or you guys through any more of this."

"She'd rather you be here in any way she can have you."

"But still, I'm giving him until Christmas to decide on a miracle."

"I think it will take a little longer than that."

"He's got until Christmas to figure this out or I'll take care of it."

28. Our Time

We never particularly cared for baseball. Or any sport for that matter. But when I was ten and suggested the two of us play catch, my dad purchased me the best glove he could afford. The leather was soft, and my fingers slid perfectly into it. He played with a glove he owned when he was a kid, but never really used.

Our first trial was in the street in front of our house.

"So how do we do this?" I asked. He shrugged.

"I think Grampie said two fingers on the laces." He threw the ball in a wide arc and the ball landed in my glove with a snap.

"We did it!" I shouted back to him.

He smiled and said, "I guess we did." We'd successfully executed this new ritual.

My throw back to my old man wasn't as graceful; it came up short and he had to chase it down into the ditch.

"Car!" I shouted. We moved out of the way for the passing car and returned to our positions on the asphalt. The afternoon went on this way for a while—his throws graceful, mine erratic and off the mark. But the sound of the ball catching in the mitt was crisp, like a message from my dad down the street safely delivered into my hand.

After an hour or so I declared I had enough, and we worked our way to the house.

"Want to watch the clouds?" he asked. Of course I did. There was nowhere in the world better than being tucked in my dad's arm watching the wispy white clouds traverse the sky. "The best part of a baseball glove is when you're done—it makes a heck of a pillow."

So we laid in the grass, our gloves resting beneath his head, mine nestled in the crook of his arm, for the rest of the afternoon. We named the cloud shapes and called out jet planes too far away to hear, their paths revealed only by their contrails. The summer air was warm, but there was a cool tinge to the constant breeze that made Pa's arms even better, like a den, safe and protected.

It wasn't long before my eyes closed, and the sun unknowingly crept across the sky, leaving me with nothing but the echoes of the glove's snap and the heat of my dad's body.

29. New Year

It was strange knowing your best friend would die in the upcoming year. New Year's Eve has always been saddled with sadness—regrets from the previous year—but at midnight that slate is always wiped clean: we kiss our loved ones and celebrate 365 days of possibility in which to set right all that went off course the prior year. But that year I struggled to understand how to approach a year with the burden of death—it would have been two years, the average for ALS patients, and unfortunately my dad was right on schedule.

Stacie, Kai and I spent the holiday at my parents' house, as we did most every year. I never liked going out on that night, as I worried about drunk drivers navigating the roads. The lighting in my parents' house was dim—a few candles and the flicker of the TV. Mom made dinner, and the high point of the evening was to be flambéed apples. My dad was too tired to come into the kitchen to watch the lighting of the fruit, but insisted we keep him updated "just in case your mother sets the house on fire and you have to roll me out of here."

Since it was quiet in the home that year, Mom set up a video chat with her cousin Jim, whom my parents had just visited in California. Mom had us position the computer far enough away from the kitchen counter so the screen wasn't set ablaze. Mom counted down from ten and flicked the lighter. Nothing. She flicked it again. "Sonofabitch," she muttered. Kai played with his cars in the living room at my dad's feet.

"Boooo," came the voice from the computer screen. "What a disappointment," said her cousin.

She flicked the lighter a few more times, then said, "Who wants rum-soaked apples?" Stacie and I raised our hands. It didn't matter, because somehow it was all okay. We were there together—lucky to live not only in the same city, but the same neighborhood as my folks. We were blessed to have these moments. Even though Pa was tired, he remained awake until midnight. We all shouted and yelled when the sparkling ball fell on TV. Kai cried when Mom blew a horn, and then giggled when Pa covered his ears to commiserate with his grandson. I kissed Stacie, Kai, Mom, then leaned into Pa. His shoulders were bone. Flesh thin. But I still kissed a warm cheek. And somehow it was okay.

30. Leaks

"I don't know what to do because I don't know how to do it myself and she was so fucking mean—the way she looked and talked to me—and she just kept making me feel like a fool. A goddamn fool." The whole stream of words from Mom was laced with tears.

I switched the phone to my left ear so I could drive with my right hand. "Mom, slow down, what happened?" She explained how the woman at the local plumbing and kitchen store that we hired to complete all our remodeling just stared at her when Mom asked for a removable showerhead to clean my dad. For every cleaning Mom had to shoulder Dad's weight, pulling him upright and sliding him to a shower seat using a transfer board. The step into the bathtub was too high for my dad and they worried he'd hurt himself badly if he attempted it. But she needed a way to shut the water off, get the stream closer, to make less of a mess in the bathroom—water spraying everywhere. She said the woman just shrugged and turned away.

"I told her I needed it. I didn't have a choice because if I couldn't get the angle just right he freezes. He just sits there and freezes. I told her his muscle was gone and he couldn't even shiver to get warm, so he just suffers. And the fucking bitch just stared at me and said she didn't know what to tell me."

I'd never heard her like this. She was hysterical. Mom usually held it together, so this was beyond unusual. And the coldness of this salesperson astounded me. "I told Penny, because her husband works with them all the time, too, and he called and yelled at the woman, but I seriously don't know what to do."

"I'll meet you at Home Depot. I'm near there. We'll find something. I'll install it—not a big deal."

"But this isn't your problem. I don't want you to have to do anything."

"Literally the easiest plumbing job ever. I'm driving there right now. If you don't show up, then I'll be angry because it will be a waste of my time."

So we met, and I wrapped my arms around her in the parking lot. I realized I hadn't hugged her in a long time. Her body felt strong, especially juxtaposed to the bones that I embraced when I held my dad. Inside we found a quality shower head, and she agreed to meet me at her house so I could install it. I'd be a few minutes, I told her, because I had to run an errand first.

"Where's Bonnie?" I shouted. I didn't wait to make it to the desk in the back of the store. A few customers turned to look at the clamor I was making. "Bonnie. I need to speak with Bonnie." By the time I made it to the back desk, the owner, a kind man who did an amazing job on our kitchen renovation the year before, was approaching me from the showroom, extending his hand for a handshake.

"It's good to see you again," he said.

"I need to speak with Bonnie—who is she?"

A middle-aged woman with curly black hair slinked from behind the supply shelves—her head first, then the remainder of her body. The owner pointed to the woman, and I stormed the desk. She flinched back and whispered a quiet, "May I help you?"

"There was a woman who came in here today looking for help—a showerhead. Does that sound familiar?"

She nodded and began to speak, but I wouldn't have it.

"All she wanted was some help. Her husband, my dad, is dying. He will be dead before the end of the year. He can't bathe himself. He is wasting away right now, gasping as we're breathing. And my mother, the woman you treated with such indifference today, came in looking for a moment of peace. She's turned to no one, not a single person, for help in any of this…and today she did. She turned to you to help her find a goddamn showerhead to ease some pain and what did you do? You treated her like she was out of her mind. Like shit."

"But I didn't know what she was asking for…"

"It doesn't matter. It doesn't matter what you didn't understand—you should have found out. You should have had the patience to help her, but you didn't. You made her feel helpless and more lost than she did when she came in."

Bonnie began to blink hard. The owner was frozen to my left. The customers had gathered at this point behind me. "What do you want? Yeah, that's what I did. What do you want from me? You want me to quit? You want me to walk out of here and quit? Because I'll quit." The owner showed no sign of emotion, but he stared at her. Hard. His eyes didn't move from her.

"That's too easy," I said. "I just want you to know that today you made someone's life worse. You made a woman who is desperately trying to hold onto every second with her dying husband fall deeper into the darkness of life. You did that. When you go to bed tonight I want you not to be able to close your eyes until you think of her trying to keep her dying husband warm in a shower. That's what I want."

My fist must have punched the counter because later that night it hurt. And I must have exited the store, and people must have stared, but I don't remember how I turned, what they looked like, or how the door opened. But I found myself in my car in the parking lot, shaking, breathing harder than I ought to. I often leave situations feeling unfulfilled, like there was another thought or word I should have said. But I felt complete. I felt like for once it came out just as it should have. It wasn't until the drive home that I worried about Bonnie, hoping she was strong enough to handle it. I hoped her husband hadn't just left her, hoped her family was healthy. I didn't know her life any more than she knew Mom's. I hoped this wasn't the final push that might spur her to end it all when she closed her eyes at night.

I entertained those thoughts only for a few miles, then resigned myself to the notion that she deserved it. That sometimes it was necessary to push back against those small moments, infractions, if it meant selfishly making your own world right for an evening.

Mom already knew when I made it to her house.

"What did you say to her?" she asked, as I stood in her shower with the old showerhead removed.

"No idea what you're talking about."

"I know you went up there."

I wrapped plumber's tape around the exposed pipe, prepping it for the new showerhead.

"It's done. Just let it be."

"You don't have to protect me, you know? I just had a bad day."

"And you didn't need it to be any worse." I stepped out of the shower and turned the handle. Hot. Cold. I detached the head, showing Mom how to stop the stream and adjust the flow. I hated that she needed this. And I hated that her home would need repairs. In a few weeks her kitchen sink would start leaking. These two worked their whole lives and gave me everything I ever needed, and I thought at this point in their lives things should be easy. That's how the commercials advertise it—retirement is when you can just call a plumber from your beach house in South Carolina to fix showerheads and dripping faucets. But they didn't have that kind of money, and now Mom was in charge of the whole ship.

"Thank you," she said.

"You're not alone in this," I said.

She nodded, took the showerhead, flicked it on, and washed any of the dirt I'd left down the drain.

31. Sequences

After years of dreaming he was paralyzed, Pa continued to have fantastic dreams where he could walk. Since he was young he'd lose the use of his legs, arms at night. The rest of the world would come alive in magic colors, but he'd sit in the room, unable to participate or move.

"And now I can walk," he explained again. "Just like that. After sixty years of being paralyzed in my dreams they went and switched on me." He looked healthier than I'd seen him in some time. There was a bit more color in his cheeks and his voice was confident. It seemed he was able to move his jaw with more strength, punch out the words with even a hint of joy.

I didn't tell him of the dream sequences I'd been having as of late. He and I would be somewhere, subway stations, malls, always throngs of people bustling about. He couldn't really walk, but instead he pulled his body along this metal rail with chipped white paint. In every dream it was the same identical rail, and the people would bump into him, not noticing his legs dangling behind his body. I pushed them, but I didn't want him to notice. I never wanted him to think he wasn't moving successfully along these paths on his own. Night after night I'd shoulder these people away from my dad, hoping we'd make it wherever we were going. But we never did.

I kept my nights to myself and just listened to his stories of newfound dream freedom.

For him the places, the scenes were the same as before—the cliffs of his hometown Fécamp, the hallways of work, his yard, but instead of idly watching, frozen, he moved around these spaces at night. "It's a nice change," he said. "It's nice to be alive somewhere."

32. Practice

People started dying. A lot of them. Floods of notices. Wakes. Funerals. So-and-so's friend. This student's grandparent. My cousins' grandma on the other side. People just kept dying. Or maybe they always had been, but I just failed to notice.

The first funeral I attended was for the dad of one of my buddies at work. Jim had told me about his dad's decline, his fight with cancer making him weaker. Then losing that fight. Despite hearing about the loss of so many other people, I know why I chose this one to attend. Of course because he was a good friend, but it was more selfish than that. Jim was just slightly older than me and had an older sister. I never had the gumption to ask how old his dad was, but his dad would be the closest in age to my dad. This wake was a test run. I had to know what a middle-aged man looked like in the casket. Not a grandma who lived a full life. But I needed to know what life-cut-short looked like, the color drained and the family robbed of the expectation of life's full arc.

The line ran out the door. Jim was a popular guy and his sister was a prominent figure in the Cleveland business scene. I went by myself because we had no one to watch Kai since Mom's time was always occupied with my dad. Jim's family stood in a line after the casket. Some guests knelt to pay their respects. The room was loud. I heard someone behind me say, "My son loves crab legs." Two boys sitting in the chairs balanced Sacajawea coins on their pointed fingers. Flowers flanked the room, reds and yellows spilling from vases. The line lumbered along. There was a board of photos on the far side of the room, thumb-tacked stills of Jim's dad, moments of laughter caught forever. A video played on a small TV in the back of the funeral home—photos put to music. The din of the room was too loud to make out the lyrics, and the television was too small to make out the details from my vantage point. It all ended up like this: red carpeting and a few dozen photos bordered by flowers to the soundtrack of unidentifiable songs. All of it. Our childhoods, ideas, interactions, creations. Our moments of love and joy and pain. This was how life concluded—a conversation about crab legs and a coin precariously placed on the tip of an index finger.

And the line lumbered on.

As I approached, I could see his dad's hands, an arm. But not his face, still no indication of his age. The man in front of me stood up, made the sign of the cross, and proceeded to greet the family. I moved slowly to the casket, but went straight to the face. He wasn't young. Clearly he wasn't a man who lived all of his days, but he wasn't my dad. The skin was too wrinkled, more breaths creased his face. His grandkids were in school, could tell stories about the time he...and when they all... His death was heartbreaking, too soon, but he wasn't the age where people move both hands to their mouths, intake a quick breath, whispering "My God" when they hear the news. Or maybe he just looked that way because he wasn't mine.

We think we're guaranteed something. Seventy-eight still feels young. The eighties are acceptable. And the nineties are when we'd like to go. That's the storyline we expect. And when that arc falls considerably short there is a disturbance to the whole matrix. My grandfather underwent quadruple bypass heart surgery a few weeks after this funeral, and I may have said, "That's unfortunate," when I found out. And better yet, when he survived the demanding surgery we felt lightened, because it's not to be expected—a pleasant surprise the old man made it. But when you're sixty and unable to support your own weight because your muscles have deteriorated to nothing because the neurons in your brain start dying one by one by one, well, that's not the course. That's not in the previews.

I lingered too long at the casket. I could feel the line's impatience as it scuffed its feet on the red carpeting. So I pursed my lips, moved to the family, shook Jim's hand and hugged him, saying something about condolences. Those words seemed to fit the room. I told him we'd talk about it more at lunch—somewhere where you could discuss the dead or the dying without red carpeting squelching life.

The remainder of the afternoon rested on the soft bands of light that soaked through the living room window. We assembled at Pa's feet, touching his legs, telling him we loved him. He smiled more than he had in months. Kai stumbled around his feet, hugging his legs, shouting, "Car," whenever one passed, just like the two of them spent their time for the past two years. When I'd dismiss myself to sob in the kitchen, Kai would follow, saying, "No cry. Don't cry, Daddy. Happy," like my dad somehow spoke through him.

Pa switched out his full-face mask to talk. He comforted us, telling us each how much he loved us. He said, "I'm happy, no offense to you guys, but I'm happy to go." I cried into his leg, clinging onto the day. The worst was to know. To know that this was the day your father would die. In the next few hours this person who raised you, this person who you trusted with your very being, would pass. To choose the words, the right words, so there were no regrets. No should haves. No I mighthavesaids. I worried what I'd say when the day came. But it was simple: "I love you." There were a few more words—how I'd miss him. How he made me the man I am and will be. But the only word that mattered that day from any of us was *love*. The word we humans have been whispering for ages. This simplicity helped to control the chaos. Love helped keep understanding in moments of misunderstanding. To be able to say it, mean it, and know that in whatever the forever of death is, infinite blackness or a golden strand pulled from the sky, it all comes down to that thing. *Love.*

"Change the oil in the lawnmower," he gasped.

"What?" I responded. I was nestled at his feet. Mom, Stacie and Kai were in the kitchen preparing lunch.

"Five things," he said. "Only five things."

"Oil is one of them?" I asked, laughing.

He nodded. "Don't fuck up my lawnmower." The adrenaline of the day made his voice robust, like maybe he shouldn't die today. His mouth couldn't make the curve of a laugh, but his eyes did, louder than any gut-driven laughter I've ever heard.

"Get a new house. Don't get stuck. We got stuck. Don't inherit someone else's problems. Ever." He breathed in hard through his nose. "Take care of your mother. She'll be fine. She's strong. But I love her. Care for her if she needs you."

I started crying.

"Stop it. And quit worrying. I worried about everything. My whole life. I always worried. And look." He blinked his eyes hard. "Look where any of it got me. Here. Not worth it. Love life. Live it. Stop worrying."

I looked up and he smiled. I don't know how he did, the muscle gone, but he smiled. "And I love you," he said. "I love you." Repeated. Even though there was nothing left.

33. Breathing Easier

Their house began to fill with contraptions. Pa was still able to shuffle about the home with the support of a walker, but his thighs were weak, preventing him from standing upright from a sitting position. The ALS Association truly took over where the doctors failed. Mom tried time and time again to gather information from the hospital on how to make Pa physically comfortable; she needed help figuring out how to complete simple tasks, like lifting him from the chair without hurting his thinning sides. Every call with the clinic ended the same: some referrals to someone else, who recommended some other department, who didn't really know. It was as if my dad was their first case of ALS, though the doctors still were able to make their monthly calls to see if my dad would be driving downtown so they could run some more tests and "gather more data for their research."

It was about that time that the future quit mattering. My younger cousin participated in the ALS walk, raising hundreds of dollars for research, but our small clan stopped looking that far ahead. The others, the next ones, didn't seem to matter because the one that counted the most to us was fading. If the doctors couldn't, or rather, refused to help find comfort, we saw no obligation to help them, or anyone else, with their papers.

So Mom entrenched herself in the blogs and online support groups for ALS caregivers. She became close friends with a woman whose online name was Rose Hope. She talked about Rose Hope (always using both names) often, like a friend, even though the two had never met. Rose's husband didn't have ALS, but another neurological disease that mimicked the symptoms of Pa's. They commiserated, cried, shared all they could. There was comfort for Mom when the hospitals stopped supporting.

In addition to the emotional ties Mom forged online and the advice from the forums, the ALS Association drove over anything Mom asked for, gifts from those who passed. In her weekly visit, Lisa from the association offered my dad a BiPAP machine—a small generator-looking device that offered additional air for my dad's lungs. In a prior visit he mentioned how it was becoming difficult to breathe, especially at night when his body was worn out. Since my dad refused to consider the option of being *trached* ("that isn't living," he said), this machine with its mask that covered the nose and mouth would provide that extra breath so my dad could be more comfortable and not strain so much.

"But once I start using it, there is no going back," Pa said. Lisa agreed. She said his body would, in fact, become more reliant on the machine, so the old man put it off for weeks, the BiPAP resting quietly on the floor next to his chair. Finally, one night after Pa's breathing became so labored that he was almost gasping, Mom suggested they try it. Lisa had showed her how to attach the mask, ensuring there was a seal to Pa's face, and flip on the machine. If the suction wasn't right, the machine would beep a warning. Mom said he smiled as soon as the air began flowing and gave her a thumbs up. The machine made loud puffing sounds, but it soon became the white noise of the evening. Pa was upset he had to rely on it at first, but after the first night of using the machine he said he hadn't slept that well in a year. "It's just that extra push that I need." Although he'd eventually rely on the machine for most hours of the day, in the beginning he only requested it in the late evening, when his muscles were scraped thin.

The machine was tough to see at first, especially because it separated him even more. He couldn't really talk when the mask was on, but could only pantomime his words. But we were all relieved it offered him some much-deserved peace in an otherwise restless day.

The bathroom became the next hurdle for Mom, as Pa could no longer hoist himself up from the chair or toilet. So the ALS Association brought her a generator-driven inflatable pillow that Pa sat on in his chair, giving him enough leverage to stand and a "toilet ejector" that sprung Pa off the commode when he was done.

"You're going to shoot me into the shower door," Pa said, watching her assemble the unit in the living room. I offered several times to help screw it together, but she wouldn't have it. She couldn't accept help from any of us. I think she didn't want to burden us, but more so, I believe she was protecting my dad. She didn't want him to feel that sense of vulnerability. He was surrounded with the safety of her eternal commitment, so he never felt like any of us were put out.

"Goddammit," she cursed, the screwdriver slipping from her hand. "God. Damn. It."

"Let me try," I said.

"No, just go home and be with your family," she said.

"Mom, I'm not going home right now, so you might as well let me try."

"No, I have to get it myself." The screwdriver slipped again. "Fuck. Fuck. Fuck." She'd been kneeling before the toilet ejector, but now put her head on the floor. She began crying, picked up the screwdriver and threw it across the living room. My dad looked at her and closed his eyes. He nodded at me. I picked up the screwdriver, patted Mom's side, indicating she should move over, and worked the screw into the toilet ejector.

"Nothing is easy anymore," she said, picking up her head. "I need to be able to fix this thing."

"But maybe not today," I said. I finished the job and returned the ejector to the bathroom, testing it out to ensure it worked. By the time I returned, Mom was cuddled on my dad's lap and the two of them were watching *Modern Family* on TV. My dad was laughing through his mask and Mom wrapped her arms around his neck, her eyes now dry, but swollen. I sat on the couch to watch the show with them when my dad let out a forceful laugh from behind his mask, causing the seal to break and the BiPAP to scream its warning. They both starting laughing hysterically at the "pop" the mask made when my dad laughed.

The show ended, and as she was resetting the machine, resealing the mask around his face, she tossed the remote into his lap and said, "Turn on the Olympics—let's see what's cooking." My dad stopped watching the TV and turned his head to her, eyes open wide. "What?" she asked. My dad tapped his mask, indicating he wanted it removed. She shook her head and removed the mask. The machine wailed.

"What did you say?" he asked, truly looking confused.

"I said, 'Turn on the Olympics—let's see what's cooking.'"

My dad tilted his head back in laughter, unable to speak. Mom cocked her head and scrunched her eyebrows at me. He couldn't stop. Finally he regained his composure and said, "I thought you said, 'Get that limp dick out—let's see what's cooking.'"

She joined his hysterics and sat back into his lap, their eyes welling with laughter. I slipped out of the room unnoticed and put on my shoes to return home. As I locked the door all I could hear was the faint ruckus of the wailing BiPAP, muffled by the roar of their laughter.

34. Funny Thing About the Disease...

Mom opened the kitchen door, hauling in groceries from the car. I'd been visiting with Pa and asked if she needed help. She said to just "keep the old man entertained." Mom was constantly in motion. She was forced to continue working to support them, but the moment she returned home she was greeted by another full-time job with no breaks. She shopped. She cleaned. She was a researcher for cures and a nurse tending to my dad's needs, but he never asked for much. He'd recently recounted a story of her washing him in the shower. She assisted him onto the seat and then washed him because he couldn't hold a washcloth or move his arms where they needed to go. "She was yelling at me about something and while she was yelling she started scrubbing my balls harder the more she got worked up. Hurt like crazy," he said, laughing. I suggested one of those golf-ball washers, and he laughed so hard he needed his BiPAP put on. But her frustration was real. Justified. She was tired. But she never stopped. Ever. Indefatigable, she'd start another day: working, cleaning, tending, but never complaining. At least he was still there. Although there was a direct correlation between the amount of profanity she used and her level of frustration, she never bemoaned her life.

"Tell your mom to come in here," Pa said one evening. "I'm getting tired. I need my machine."

Mom had heard him, and without my saying came into the living room. "You're a real pain in the ass," she said, laughing. He stuck out his lower lip. She started up the machine and strapped the mask to his face. She did it with the ease of a seasoned caregiver. The way her hands slipped the contraption over his head was gentle.

Pa tried to mouth something to me, but I couldn't make out the words. He did it again, but still nothing. Pa tapped the mask. His fingers were beginning to permanently bend. "Pain in the ass," she said, smiling. When Pa tapped the mask there was either a problem with the seal or he needed it removed. She slipped it off.

"Be sure to check that valve under the sink to make sure it's not dripping," he said. His voice was exhausted. Mom slipped it back on.

He tapped it again. Mom looked at him and shook her head. "Last time," she said. Pa breathed hard. He said I needed to check the oil in the lawnmower, and began to rattle off instructions of how to check some valve on the weed whacker to make sure it wasn't leaking.

"I say put the mask back on," I said. Mom laughed and did just that, cutting my dad off midsentence.

My dad waved his hands around, and mouthed, very clearly even through the mask, "What. The. Heck?" She continued tightening the straps (maybe even a tug too tight) to secure the seal. She gave him a light slap on the head and went back into the kitchen, laughing all the way.

The body was crumbling to ash, yet, there was still laughter. So much laughter.

35. Dream Sequence Two: With More Frequency

Pa rode down a snow-covered hill between Stacie and me on a red, plastic disc sled. We were out of control, the trajectory heading us into trees and snowdrifts, but we bounced like a pinball, ricocheting back onto the course. All the while we soared, my dad couldn't speak or communicate, but as we went whirring down the hill he smiled a wide, toothy grin, only mouthing the words, "Faster, faster," the sled obeying his every command.

36. Sold

I don't remember when he drove his car for the final time. There was no "this is it" or "I can't." He simply backed it into his spot in the garage between the hanging ladder and the snow blower, and worked his way out of the car. He continued to drive much longer than he could freely walk. Still able to press the gas and brake quickly, it surely enabled him to feel part of the world a little bit longer. When we'd meet them in Rocky River, a perfect little park with swings and benches that overlooked a scenic Lake Erie beach, he'd often park the car and begin walking the relatively short distance down the steep hill to the base of the park where the majority of the benches resided, his walker offering him breaks down the walk of a few dozen feet. With time and decay, he'd remain at the top of the hill, gazing out at the crashing waves and kids playing in the sand. And I remember the day he said he'd just stay in the car and watch, because it hurt too much to be pulled out of the driver's seat and work his way the few feet to the rail. "I can see just fine from here," he said. "I'm just glad to be here."

Eventually his car had been stagnant in the garage for months. I drove it to work one day when my van was in the shop for repairs. I sat in the seat and turned over the engine; it sputtered, yet came alive on the first crank. The dashboard clock was off an hour. He always reset it the day the time changed because he had no patience for a clock being off. But there it sat, an hour off, the last time he'd sat in the seat. So I reset the clock and turned on the radio, which immediately went to a Gary Moore CD that he'd been listening to the last time he'd been in there. The whole experience felt holy, like wandering around the wreckage of Pompeii, everything left as it was in those final moments. The guitar howled on the CD, mournful notes being wrenched from the belly of the guitar—how he loved the blues. The Lackeys were still coming around nearly every week to share wine and cheese with my folks, filling their days with stories outside of the house. David said he and my dad should start playing the slide guitar. "You don't have to use your fingers," he said. "Just move the slide up and down the neck." Pa explained to David his new aversion to music, except French songs. When he wasn't watching movies he listened to French radio. He couldn't explain it, but it was the only music that was tolerable. Maybe it was a return to something hopeful since his childhood home and the ocean were too far away.

It wasn't long after I borrowed the car that I asked Mom what we were going to do with it. I invited her to lunch at an outdoor wine bar on a warmer winter day just to get her out of the house for some time; her head seemed to get heavier by the day. "It's just sitting there losing money," I said. I knew she hated to talk about money or more work. "I can do it for you—take it in and see what I can get for it."

"No, I know. It's the right thing to do," she said. She took a sip of wine. "It's good." She nodded to the glass. I stayed quiet. "It just feels really final, you know? But you're right, he can't drive. He won't ever drive or even really move again."

"I can do it if it's too hard for you. Each one of these things becomes another symbol, another transition to the end. But it's a hybrid and those batteries probably need to run and if they go, you won't get anything for the car."

She was quiet for a moment and took another sip of wine. "It just sucks." Her eyes welled. "It just all, sucks." I could barely hear her last words because she tucked them into her throat. "We drove to Nova Scotia in that car. When he bought it, he figured a hybrid would be good because we were retiring soon and we'd take it everywhere. Anywhere we wanted. We'd run it into the ground, he said. I didn't think he'd be gone before the car."

I reached out for her hand and she cried. And we drank. And I eventually broke the silence. "Let's go together. Tomorrow. I'll make an appointment."

"I'll make it," she said, interrupting me.

"Fine, you make it and we'll go together. It's just a car. Wheels, oil and an engine." And movement. His last stab at movement.

She nodded and we drank our wine and cried and laughed and felt the warm sun burn the tops of our heads.

We went the next day and received a more-than-fair price. The man at the dealership said the car looked like it had never been driven. Mom said her husband waxed it every other week and cared for it like a baby. "It shows," he said. "We'll have no problem selling this."

After they wrote her a check, she opened the trunk before handing over the keys to make sure she had everything. We'd already retrieved a small little robot with magnetic feet that I gave to my dad when I was five. He used to have it hanging from the ceiling of his pickup truck, and then subsequently transferred it to every car he ever owned. It reminded him of me, he said.

But there was nothing left in the car. The glove compartments were emptied and hands were swept under the seats to check for anything that might have been lost. The dealer handed her my dad's plates, "144 Volts," a custom plate my dad ordered for the number of volts in his hybrid car. She handed the man the keys, closed her eyes, and as we left she traced her hand over the hood of the car and down the trunk, patting it slightly like a friend or a past or a future that was leaving forever.

37. More Tests

He raised his right hand, and said, “Half an inch.” He tried to put his thumb and pinky together. They were half an inch apart. He lacked the muscle to get them closer. He tried again. “Half an inch. Half an inch.” His hand fell to his lap.

38. New Lows

Somehow a week passed. A week and I hadn't seen him or touched his arm. We had been busy with work and Kai. We spoke every day on the drive home from work, and he sounded strong, or at least better. When you're not there to witness the decay, it's easy to conjure up flesh, muscle and breath. Regeneration. Myths. He told all sorts of brief stories in that week. The movies spurred memories from his youth—the time he and a cousin dug a fort into the side of a hill (the top covered with a layer of grass) so they could smoke cigarettes without getting caught.

He said he loved the sea. Growing up in Fécamp, France, ocean side, he'd always had an affinity for water. When he was twelve and initially came to the States, the first purchase he made was a small boat to sail around the quarries in Berea, Ohio. He said he'd bring friends along if they'd ask, but he preferred the quietness of the lake, the wind his only mode to move. As his disease progressed he began looking up boats on the Internet. Since his days consisted of Netflix movies and YouTube clips, he liked to explore all kinds of things. I never asked him why a boat. "Not sure what I'd get," he told me one day on the drive home. "There is something nice about a big sailboat, but those little guys, the Flying Dutchman, I think that's what I'll get when I get better. Take it out and just go." This was the only time I'd heard him speak of a future in months, especially a future that wasn't bleak and riddled with sadness. I nodded and agreed that would be nice. He told me what it used to be like on the ocean. We talked about our vacation back to Fécamp nearly fifteen years prior, when he showed me the beaches he used to comb for treasures and the spot the people from the village would stand to welcome back the fishermen after they'd been out to sea for months hauling in their catch. "Maybe I just want a boat because it reminds me of being a kid. I liked being on the water. I always did." He never mentioned the boat with the slightest bit of irony. He just kept repeating how a boat would be nice when he got better. "Just being out there felt safe and calm," he said. I think he now wanted to get back to that place, in a boat, able to harness and control the wind, instead of being at the mercy of nature.

He only mentioned it that day, and never again. It was like he allowed himself to go somewhere else for a time to escape the entombment that was cementing him into the chair.

Those stories provided some kind of optimism. Not seeing him in person, but hearing the strong timber of his voice made me believe there was a way out of the whole mess. That maybe he could get better and start to believe in dreams again.

But then I stopped over with Kai. His cheeks were sinking into his jaw and he'd lost so much weight his eyes looked too large for his face. His gauntness was evident everywhere, his thin wrists, his sweatpants hanging off his thighs like loose skin.

Kai ran to his lap and hugged his knees. "Papa!" Kai adored his grandfather. Pa slowly reached his hand out and rested it on Kai's head. "My boy," he said, smiling.

Even though I knew the answer, I asked him how it was going.

"Not good," he said. "Something is happening again. I'm hot and then really cold, and I can't breathe. Even just sitting here is an effort."

Kai retrieved a few cars from the play pen and said, "Up?" He always played on my dad's lap. He didn't really know a mobile grandfather. This was the version he knew, and he loved him without restraint.

I asked my dad if it was okay to put him on his lap, and he said,

"Sure." Kai nestled into his body, running the cars up and down his arms like highways.

"There's no cure on the horizon," he said. "You know that." I nodded.

Mom came into the room and sat down. "I asked him about the trach, but he wouldn't even talk about it."

"To what end?" he asked. His voice was strong. "So I can just sit here and waste away longer?" But only for the moment, as it trailed into something weaker. "It's just not worth it."

Mom sighed.

Pa used whatever strength he had to pull Kai close to him. Kai smiled and ran the cars over Pa's head and down his chest. "Love you," Kai said.

"I love you. Always." We sat in the silence for a bit. "Did you get rid of that table yet in your living room?"

"Not yet," I said. "We will this weekend."

"Tonight. When you go home, get rid of that stupid thing. I told you—I was watching the news and if it's not shatter-proof glass and Kai smacks it just right and puts him arm through it, he'll rip his muscles to shreds. And..." His voice waned again. He couldn't sustain it.

This turn was hard. I worried about Mom, what this new phase must be like for her, each a new beginning toward an ending. Each turn surely hurt more.

Pa tried to adjust, but he didn't have the strength to push himself up in his seat. He was always more tired at the end of the day. "I want to die," he said.

"Not today," Mom said. "I just made dinner and it would be a waste not to eat it." He smiled.

"No, seriously, we put Eddie down at this point," he said. "It's just the right thing to do." After a tumor showed up on their dog's neck, they let her live out her final days until she grew uncomfortable. Then my dad coerced her to the car with treats and drove her to the vet, stroking her back while the pentobarbital worked through her body.

"What should I do," Mom asked, "lead you to the car with some wine and cheese?"

Pa laughed. "Yes, that would be a fine way to go."

Mom stood up to head into the kitchen when Kai leapt off of Pa's lap and ran to Mom, smacking her on the butt. This action was so out of character for him, but he burst into high-pitched laughter and did it again. Mom giggled. He then turned and saw Pa struggling to stand to adjust himself in the seat. His arms gave out twice. Kai pointed and began laughing again. "Papa is so funny," he said. Kai started imitating my dad's awkward motions and Pa began laughing so hard, he was running out of breath. He was gasping, head tilted back to get air. I thought for a moment he may actually laugh himself to death, and I thought maybe that would be okay. That might be a fine way to go.

Kai ran back to my dad and climbed into his lap. He wrapped his arms around his neck and said again, "You are funny."

Mom smiled and went into the kitchen, and Kai settled back into play.

"It's not dying, you know," Pa said.

"What do you mean?" I asked.

"I'm not scared of dying, I'm scared of living. Horrified of what might happen—all frozen, unable to move anything but my eyes. Scares the hell out of me."

He'd been speaking too much. He tired himself out. He began gasping. I jumped up and pulled Kai from his lap. He sucked in his cheeks for air, like a fish, trying to be something, anything at all.

"Mom," I called. "He needs his mask." She said she'd be right there.

While we waited for her, Pa refused to take a break. He had things to say today. Maybe he knew how hard it would soon be to say the most simple things. "I spent my whole life worrying, kid. My whole life. Everything—about you, Mom, my job, if I was doing anything in my life right." He breathed. "It's not worth it. You can't worry like I did.

Because where did it get me? Right here. Nothing changes because of worrying. Promise me." He paused. "Promise me you'll just live and let everything slip off. It's not worth it because in the end. In the end we all end up here. Our stories all end the same way. The difference is how we get there."

Kai played at his feet, tickling them with his cars. He smiled.

Mom dried her hands on a towel and threw it over shoulder. She flicked the machine on. "I love you," he said, right before she slipped the mask onto his face.

"I love you, too."

I told Kai it was time to go. He hugged my dad, and he gave the best hug back he could give. Mom returned to the kitchen and Pa's breathing began to return to normal, evenly paced breaths. As we left the room I looked back to see his eyes were closed and his head was down, like he was dead or praying or maybe imagining himself on a boat, pulling into the dock to the cheers of hundreds of French children, a hero returning home.

*I found Mom pacing in the backyard. It was cold, but she wasn't wear-*ing a coat. She said, "We're going to need to plan something. A party. I don't want a funeral."

"Not today," I said. "We don't have to think about that right now." Her eyes were red. There was no more for them to give.

"I want food and wine and a party. We need a movie. Something better than what everyone else does."

"I'll do it."

"We could show that video he made of himself." My dad made a montage of still pictures set to music for everyone in the family. He began compiling the projects before electronic photos, using his VHS camera to take each image. Since he was the only one who made the videos in the family, he had to make his own—his life from France to now in black and white and then color. The last one he did.

"Would it be tacky to ask him where it is on the computer before he goes?" Mom laughed.

"We're going to be okay, you know?"

"I think that's what I worry about the most—that day when I'm okay again."

39. Saints

I'd begun to think about saints. I'd lost all connection to organized religion during college, and we were never even Catholic, but I began to understand the appeal of a person who could heal it all. Fix it. Make everything shitty in this world tolerable. The only saint my dad ever spoke about was Saint Thérèse. His Catholic upbringing had also been shed midway through his life, but for some reason she always remained. The family possessed a small scrap of her cloak, a patch of cloth in a tiny plastic bag with a card declaring its authenticity. My grandma brought it over on the boat when they immigrated to the U.S., and my dad still prayed to Thérèse every morning. When his father was dying of a brain aneurism, flown to Canada for a specialized surgery, my dad said he walked into a random church in Ontario to pray. He'd just left his father and mother at the hospital, the doctor saying he only had hours left. My dad was tired and distraught with emotion, alone in this church. And he said as he looked up he saw her, St. Thérèse, hovering before him. She was speaking without speaking, telling him to go back to the hospital. And he did. He rushed in the doors and his father's condition had changed. He turned a corner no one had expected. And within days he was sent back to the U.S. and would be home. Healthy. Alive. A miracle.

After my grandpa was in the clear, my dad drove home straight without stopping because he missed us so deeply, but when he opened his car door, he was unable to walk. Mom helped shoulder his weight into the house. He cried and told us how much he'd missed us. He brought me a silver futuristic car that moved forward after I pulled it backwards. And he cried and cried. His ability to walk soon returned, but I'd always wondered why. Was it the hours in the car that cramped his legs? Emotional exhaustion? The byproduct of the miracle? The foreshadowing of ALS?

I have always and will always struggle with the story of St. Thérèse's manifestation. My dad was no liar, nor a believer in what can't be seen. He was spiritual, but not religious. But that story, he swore, was as real as anything he'd ever known. Perhaps the mind hallucinates. Perhaps a series of events fall in line one after the other: a delirium, a fluke medical recovery, cramped legs. There is no reason why I shouldn't believe those aren't the explanations. But the story is from my dad, and he has never exaggerated. He wasn't capable. Life, he always said, is enough, there is no reason to tell stories to make it any greater.

So I struggle. I believe in St. Thérèse's connection to my father. That she came to him. That she will again. Yet that's as far as my faith will allow me to progress. I don't know about a god or spirit or even another saint. But I believe in that afternoon in that church in Ontario. And there are days when I turn to that connection for hope, not for me or humanity or religion, but for my dad alone. For his sake. Because that's enough.

We all called upon the story of Thérèse during my dad's decline. I suppose we all wanted another miracle. The story. A moment when she would come to me in a dream and we find my father walking and breathing like before. But that is the stuff of movies and bad books. Miracles only seem to come when there is a chance, an old man in a hospital who could recover. Not a middle-aged man with a terminal disease. Not even the saints can cure the helpless. During a conversation one day my dad asked what I thought happened when it was all over. I told him I honestly had no idea. "It's all pretty scary," he said. "When your time is up, what if it's all just blackness?" I told him he had to believe in something else.

Even if I didn't know how, I needed him to believe because he was my hope. My saint. "You know that Marissa woman I used to work with?" I nodded. "She was that born-again Christian. Anyhow, when I quit or retired or whatever I did, she asked me if I thought God had abandoned me. I laughed when she asked me, and I said 'yes.' I think the gods have left us all." I fear they were never even here, except for a saint who appeared to my father in Canada, offering him hope that maybe in the end he won't be alone. In kingdom come. On Earth as it is.

40. Calls

I'd grown gun shy of answering the phone. So many of the calls those days were bad news, panic, and tears. So when the main office patched Stacie through to my classroom while I was teaching a senior literature class, I knew something was wrong.

All I could hear were sobs. "I had to pick him up. He fell, but I need you to come home after work instead of grocery shopping because I'm not right. I'm not okay this time. He was like a car. It was like picking up a car."

"Pa or Kai?"

"Your dad. I'm sorry, your dad."

I told my students to start working on their papers. I hung up with Stacie and called her back on my cell phone in the hallway. She was still crying when she picked up.

"He fell," she began again. "He called and was breathing hard, and whispered 'I fell,' but when I asked him to repeat it he couldn't, so I ran over with Kai under my arm and I found him on the ground, flat on his back, and he was blue. And barely breathing, so somehow..." She trailed off and began to cry. I leaned against the wall outside my class, bent at the knees, pushing hard to keep myself upright. "Somehow I lifted him back to his seat. He was so heavy and Kai just sat there on the ground watching while I pulled him back to his seat." She breathed heavily.

"Are you still there?"

"No, your mom is there. I called her and she came home from work. She said I could go. I stayed a while, but it was so scary—his body just on the ground like that, you know?" She began crying again. So did I. "His body, that strong body that treated me like a dad ever since the day I met him. You can't imagine the way he looked. And I don't even know how he managed to call, to reach for the phone, because he was so weak. He said he crawled to the phone for like ten minutes, but it took all his strength and he couldn't even talk much when I answered—just heaving and breath."

My dad was still slightly mobile—he had that routine of standing twice a day while Mom was at work—once to use the bathroom, and once to shuffle into the kitchen with his walker to retrieve his lunch from the fridge. Stacie said he lost his balance when he was returning from the kitchen and as he tried to rebalance himself, find an equilibrium, his body shifted too much the other direction, causing him to spill onto the hardwood floor. He couldn't stand from his chair without assistance, so the floor was insurmountable.

Stacie said Mom was shaken up, saying she had to find a way to be home with him because "this is insane." Stacie said she just kept repeating that as she stroked his head, his breathing machine strapped on to regain some strength, or at least breathe.

I just listened. I didn't know what to say. Stacie said time was muddled—she didn't remember leaving our house with Kai or bursting into my parents' back door. It was all just an instinct of adrenaline. "His body was so heavy, yet not, you know? Like, it was hard for me to lift, but when I finally had him back in his chair and I touched his back, it was all bone—like the muscle was gone." She paused. "I haven't touched him in a long time—I'm so scared of making him uncomfortable."

I told Stacie we were lucky that she was on maternity leave and that she was home. "He could have died," I said.

"That's what he said. When I was leaving, after he recovered with his mask, he had it removed so he could tell me thank you and that he loved me. And he said he wasn't sure why he called—that maybe it would have been better if he would have just lost his breath there on the floor. Then he said he was surprised by how badly the body wants to live. Even though all he wants is to die, he didn't even think about it in that moment. He said it was as if his body fought to stay alive despite his will to die."

I heard a noise in my classroom—a student sharpening her pencil, a low clamor of voices inside the door. "I have to go," I said. I thanked her, checking once more to ensure she was okay. I hung up the phone, and reentered the classroom bustling with life.

41. Inevitables

"This is a fucking horrible way to die." I looked up to see my dad talking to Stacie.

My dad wasn't a complainer. I'd seen him lacerate his skin on metal jutting out of a bent car and work his body to exhaustion in his yard without a single objection. But this was something different.

"I know, Dan. But you are truly amazing—there is no one else who could be this strong," Stacie said.

We were at their house while I completed my parents' taxes. My mom detested numbers, so I agreed to do it for them this year since Pa couldn't hold a pen anymore. I had to break the news that they owed $2,000 to the Feds because the school my dad used to work for screwed up and didn't withhold enough money from his check. The administration wrote him an apology letter.

"That's a lot of money," Mom said. "It's just really bad timing." She looked bad. She took medical leave from work to stay home with my dad all day; he could no longer move on his own. Lisa from the ALS Association came over to show her different transfer techniques. The board she'd been using for the shower was one method, but now there was a belt she could use to hoist my dad from one place to the next. A giant bruise formed on her wrist, one of the many marks of being a constant caregiver. The transfers from the bed to the bathroom to the chair and back were tougher on my dad as of late and she had to help much more.

"It is a lot of money," I said. "Do you have enough in your checking account or do you need to transfer some?"

She said she didn't know. Pa was frustrated, trying to teach her about the numbers, but I could see it was too much today for her. She didn't need something else. Her dad was in the hospital with medical issues, her father-in-law was dying, her husband was worsening before her eyes. She didn't need another responsibility.

"You need to learn it," Pa demanded.

"It's okay," I said. "She'll get it."

Mom didn't answer.

"I'm not going to be around much longer. You have to be able to do this." I know he wanted her to be okay, or maybe he just needed to know she'd be okay.

"She'll be okay," I whispered. He nodded his head. He knew.

But I didn't. Her checks were small. She worked for over twenty years for the school district, creating innovative programs for the elementary students in her library. For twenty years she woke up every morning to instill the love of reading in children. She provided a service and a resource that was invaluable to these kids. Twenty years. But without a BA or MA or any other college degree her checks remained scant homages to real money.

"I'm worried about her," I told Stacie in private. "Without my dad's income—I don't know what that looks like."

"We can help her," Stacie said.

"But that's insane. The system should take care of her. But it doesn't give a shit about how smart or dedicated she is. It only cares about that goddamn degree."

I finished their taxes, wrote the check for my dad, and held the paperwork while he attempted a signature. It was all sketchy and abstract—not the stately signature he'd pen at the end of letters he wrote to me, even as an adult, telling me how proud he was of everything I'd become.

"What's the old joke?" he asked as he moved the pen on the paper. "Taxes and death, the two things you can count on."

I nodded. "I think that's how it goes."

"It is," he said. "That's how it goes."

42. Perfectly Normal

On February 12, 2010, Amy Bishop, a researcher at the University of Alabama in Huntsville, sat in a biology department meeting. She'd taught her anatomy and neurosciences classes early that day. A student described the lectures as "perfectly normal." The same words a fellow professor used to describe the first thirty-five minutes of the department meeting—"normal." Then at approximately 4:00 PM, CST, Dr. Bishop, who had just recently been denied tenure, pulled out a 9mm handgun and began to execute her colleagues. Three died, three others were injured.

Dr. Bishop raised the gun to her own head and pulled the trigger, but it jammed. Witnesses said she looked "perplexed." Another professor managed to push her out the door and barricade it, preventing any further casualties. No more deaths.

When Dr. Bishop was arrested outside the building, she was quoted as saying, "It didn't happen. There's no way."

Dr. Amy Bishop claimed to be on the verge of discovering a cure for ALS. The ALS forums cried conspiracy, that she found a cure, which like cancer conspiracies, say there is too much money to be made by *not* finding a cure. Though, the *New York Times* stated, "In fact, scientists who have looked at Dr. Bishop's résumé said they saw no evidence of genius, no evidence of a cure for diseases like A.L.S."

43. Birthday Gifts

March 15, 2010. Thirty-three. I used to worry about dying at thirty-three, the age Jesus died. It was just something that stuck in my head as a kid when I heard Jesus was crucified at thirty-three years old. I thought that's when I'd die, too. My estimates were right, but I was off one person.

I dropped off some chili at Mom's house. We weren't planning much of a celebration that year. It was selfishly hard with my father sitting in the corner of the room, a looming reminder of our own mortality. He wouldn't allow us to take pictures after a certain time. I'd been documenting it all along, because I feared I'd forget what his face looked like. I worried I didn't have enough pictures, but I understood his request. Why would anyone want to be remembered with sunken cheeks and bulging eyes, frail and broken?

Mom told me to run in to say hello to Pa in the living room. He was wearing his full face mask, making it impossible to communicate with words. He pointed to the table. I had no clue what he was saying. "You look like Goose in *Top Gun*," I said. He smiled big behind the mask and gave me a thumbs up. "So, happy birthday to me, right?" He smiled and mouthed something. "At the very least you could hum me a birthday song behind that thing, Goose."

He shook his head and let out a muffled laugh. "Mom still beating you up?" We'd been joking earlier in the week about Mom still being rough with him in the shower. It had little to do with how she was hurting him, but more that there was nothing left to his body but hurt. Mom walked by the living room and he mouthed something we couldn't discern. "What?" He mouthed two words again, clearly amusing himself. The suction to his mask released as he broke into laughter, the sudden whoosh of air breaking the seal. The alarm screamed and Mom came into the room to reset it.

While she readjusted the straps, he gathered himself and said, "I was saying, she sucks." Mom snapped the elastic strap against his head and he flinched. "Sorry I didn't get you anything, kiddo, for your birthday."

"Next year," I said.

He smiled, but then his eyes went down.

"Stop the sadness," Mom said. She had a way of staying upbeat, even though we all knew about next year.

"I love you, Maverick," he said.

"Well, that definitely adds a new twist to that film, but I love you, too, Goose." Mom reattached the mask and Pa went back to his silence. I kissed him on the head, and Mom walked me to the car, wishing me a happy birthday. I could see Pa through the front window and he waved, then turned his hand around and gave me the finger—ala *Top Gun.* I could see the corners of his mouth raise behind his mask—gifts when there are none to give.

44. Calls II

That's the way the calls started to come in now—moments of absolute urgency. When the phone rang at home, Mom said to hurry, run, that she needed me. As I rushed in the back door, Mom called from the bathroom. My dad was stuck on the toilet. His legs were no longer operable. That moment. He was able to get into the bathroom with her assistance, but that was the moment when his legs stopped. Forever.

The weight of his body was pushing down on nerves, causing him to black out in the bathroom. Because of the narrowness of their bathroom, Mom wasn't strong enough to both lift him and get his body out of the space. So, still wearing my jacket and shoes, I hoisted him from the side of the toilet and carried his dead weight to the hallway, where Mom had a seat with wheels waiting for him. He wasn't fully conscious. I hurried him into the living room, where Mom strapped the BiPAP to his head, both of us hoping his brain hadn't been deprived of too much oxygen.

We waited. Watched. Mom held her hand to her mouth and wept. And then the mask fogged up, Pa gasped, and his eyes opened. But no sooner had he come alive then his body began to shake like a seizure. Mom wrapped his fleece blanket around him, tucking it behind his body to cocoon him. When the convulsions ceased, he motioned for me to come near the mask. He mouthed, "Please hook the end of this hose up to the stove." He smiled. A tired smile. But a smile.

His breathing slowed to normal and he mouthed, "I'm okay."

"Compared to what?" Mom asked with a smile coupled with tears.

I let the two of them hold hands, and I called Stacie to tell her everything was okay. Or as okay as it could be. When I returned Pa said the two of us were watching him like it was his deathbed. It was. This is what death looks like.

He fought to free his hand from the blanket and held it out to shake mine. "I love you," he said. I said I love you back, through the tears.

As I left, Mom said he needed a bedpan. For now. Until they could figure out this next part. But we both knew he would never walk on his own again.

A man holding an orange sports drink and another buying detailing spray for the inside of his car. These were the first two people I saw when I walked into the local drug store. The man with the sport bottle ran his hand through his thick, brown hair and he whistled. I looked up at the aisle labels suspended from the ceiling—chips, toys, elderly care. I knew that's where it would be. Elderly care. He wasn't elderly. I remained frozen at the front of the store. I didn't want to make the trip down that unfair aisle. The man continued to whistle, rifling through a magazine rack. I didn't know the song this middle-aged man was singing, but I knew, keys gripped in hand, I wanted to drive my car key through his eye into the back of his skull. I'd twist it, to make sure. I fantasized about this man dying, so happy, unknowing. I wanted everyone to suffer with me. He looked up, surely noticing me staring, unmoving from the front of the store. He nodded and smiled. I didn't react.

"Can I help you find something?" the clerk behind the counter asked. I shook my head and walked to the Elderly Care aisle. This was an aisle Mom would grow to know more and more in the upcoming weeks. Hair-washing kits, because he was too frail to make the transfer to the tub anymore. She'd use the boxed kit to at least make him feel human, washed, and clean. I studied the five different types of bedpans, unsure of the differences. Not able to spend any sort of time in this aisle without my anger festering, I bought the most expensive. I didn't know what it did or why it was so much more than the others, but if this was where we were, he would have the best available.

After dropping it off with Mom, I spent the afternoon and the next day avoiding my parents' house. I'd been able to at least cope with each new phase, but this turn was something else.

The changes came in quickly. The ALS Association still was my parents' lifeline, providing advice, materials, devices, whatever Mom asked for. They dropped off a several-thousand dollar electric wheel chair designed to contour specifically to the body of an ALS patient. It was giant, too big for my parents' house. But we thought maybe it would allow him to leave the house, into the outside he'd always loved. Mom and I talked ramps and trajectories. But he said not to waste our time—that he had no interest anymore. And each bump in the sidewalk would be hell, the jarring would be too much pain, not worth the smell of fresh air. So Mom rearranged furniture inside and we explained how this was great for Pa, how he could have some mobility back. He tried eating at the kitchen table for the first time in a year in the new chair, but the angles were off; he choked on the dinner, losing his air. His body was too far gone. "Rocks," he said. "It feels like rocks digging into my back." The seat was well cushioned, but Pa was unable to get comfortable in the device. There was only one place in the world my dad's body didn't perpetually rest in agony—the living room chair. At night, he said, the covers in bed were too heavy, even just the sheets. They weighed down on his body, causing great aching to his feet and legs. And wrinkles were the worst. Mom had to ensure the bottom sheets were completely flattened before she transferred Pa to bed, because he said each pinch of fabric cut like razors all night. Each day was hell. And with the progression of ALS, the next day would always be worse.

The hospital finally called—it had been weeks since my parents heard from them. They wanted to know his final decision on the trach. "No trach," Mom said over the phone. "He doesn't want to live that way."

I inconsiderately needed to get away. Even just for a night. My wife was asked to give a poetry reading in Pittsburgh, so we packed up the van and the three of us took a vacation. We toured the hills of the city, ate breakfast at an adorable 50s diner recommended by our friend Jen, and spent the next day at the Phipps Conservatory, where Kai clapped at the fish in the displays and took some awkward steps in the botanical garden's green space. It was only a day, but somehow I convinced myself there wasn't a world of suffering back home. "It's been a long time since I've felt like this," I said to Stacie while we ate lunch outside the conservatory.

"Like what?"

"Normal. Just a normal family. Going on trips and out to breakfast. It's really nice."

Stacie squeezed my hand. Kai giggled at the way the breeze was turning the umbrella we were sitting beneath. "I love that kid," Stacie said.

Kai had chunks of macaroni and cheese stuck to his face and Stacie wiped them off. "It's just weird when you think about Kai and my dad. Like, now Kai has surpassed my dad's physical abilities. I knew they would meet somewhere, like a graph, as my dad declined and Kai thrived. I thought about that as soon as he was diagnosed. I just didn't think it would all happen so quickly. I thought that time would stretch and give us more moments. But right now Mom is probably wiping Pa's face, too, because he can't."

Stacie nodded. "Let's just enjoy this for now. Here. It's selfish, but let's just stay away for these few more hours so we can recharge for the next few months, because I think you're right, he's declining quickly."

Kai giggled. "Umbella," he said, pointing.

Just then an older man with gray hair creeping from the edges of his khaki cap walked next to us. He pointed his cane toward Kai. "Treasure that age," he said, his voice high and strange.

Surprised, I looked up and smiled at the man rather abruptly.

"Treasure the time. All of it." He smiled at us, and before we could say a word he scuffled away, like an aged prophet, his shoes scraping on the pebbled concrete, his movements deliberate and real.

The rest of the day was business. Doctors signed off, giving the okay for a hospice nurse to come into the home and administer morphine so my dad would be unconscious, and then his mask would be removed. The phone rang. Mom responded to questions with short, terse answers. We didn't tell anyone else in the family. I asked about Grandma and everyone agreed she shouldn't know, but should come over. I picked her up—told her he was declining and that she should say what she needed to say. There was no reason to be greedy in that moment. It was her son. Pa didn't want any guests, but he understood. They said little. She talked about the weather a bit. Pa was still upbeat, so he spoke when he could through the mask. Mouthed the word "love" and accepted her kiss on his head.

"When?" I asked Mom. She didn't know. They said hospice would call an hour or so before they were coming, and then we should start the first dose of morphine to use up what was left in the house. They'd bring much more and we'd progress from there.

And so it was. We hugged my dad, circled at his legs. We held onto time any way we could, though it slipped through our fingers like oil.

Then the phone rang. Mom took it in the other room. "Un-huh. I understand. Of course. Yes, he's ready."

She came back into the room with the bag of morphine—the liquid would slip down his throat, not enough to knock him out, but at least to get it started.

Pa smiled. Moved his only working hand to his heart. And back down again.

We each said what we needed to. Our last moments before he became foggy. Before the words didn't matter much anymore, only touch and darkness. Those words are ours. Between us. Of course we said "love" over and over, but the others will always remain ours. Even Kai, wrapped in his lap for the final time. They are his. Whether or not he remembers them word for word or at all doesn't matter, but they remain something between each of us and my dad. Sacred.

Mom was the last—we gave her time. We put Kai to bed after he stretched and tip-toed to my dad to give him a kiss. "Love you, Papa," he said.

The full mask had been switched out so he could speak freely. "Love you, my kiddo," Pa said back.

The house was dark. We could hear tears and soft words between my parents. Stacie tucked Kai into bed in the back room, and I went to the garage to wait for the nurse. This was Mom's last time with her husband of forty years. She'd administer the first and second doses. I'd wait for the hospice nurse, the messenger from here to there. It was cold outside. The air felt damp even though there was no rain. I shivered, looking in the kitchen door, light filling the home. Kai was surely asleep by then, his sweet breath near Stacie's face. And Mom surely sat at Pa's feet, locked into whatever embrace she could.

There were no stars that night. Only a chill that made my breath into ghosts. A dog barked and then howled. A turn signal lit up the house across the street. Headlights cut through the darkness of the evening, slowed before Mom's driveway and turned, blinding me for a moment in a rapture of light. She was here. Her car filled with enough doses. She was here to help my dad die.

45. VooDoo

After a while all you can do is talk. Our time was spent engaged in these chats in their living room. Whenever we could steal a moment we were with him because we knew time was short. Pa always braided every conversation with humor. One day he said, "You know you have a good wife. And Kai is special—I like the way you're raising him, like an adult." I thanked him and he said, loud enough for Mom to hear, "But I don't know about that wife of mine—she jumps around here like crazy when she vacuums, no order. No nice lines like you're supposed to have."

Mom shouted from the back room, "If you don't like it, get off your ass and do it yourself." He laughed whatever he had left.

Later he told us he had a dream that God would decide that next morning whether to cure him or kill him. Mom said when he woke and she removed his mask, he said with a smile, "Fuck, I'm still alive."

He continued to track his own decline with his pinky and thumb. They didn't even come close anymore. I never knew hands contained that much muscle and fat until I saw my father's at the end—literally skin dangling from bone, sinking into the gaps where muscle used to reside. He shook his head after every test, each day worse than the next. He was running out of breath.

Mom went back to blaming herself for his disease. When he was healthy and trying to regulate his cholesterol, just prior to the diagnosis, she thought she'd given him the wrong foods that somehow triggered the malfunction. To combat this failure, she signed up with Stacie for Reiki classes at a local wellness center. Reiki is the belief that by laying hands on (or near) a person, you can heal them by transferring life force to enhance that person's physical and mental state. One can be trained in Reiki from a master who passes on the knowledge of how to transfer the life force to another, even if you're not in the same room.

"Goddamn voodoo," Pa said. "You see what this witch is doing? As if I wasn't messed up enough, now we have voodoo." Mom held out her hands toward him, fingers up, palms out. "Shoot me now." Mom giggled.

"This isn't helping the life force transfer," Mom said.

"Neither is this disease," he said. "I don't know what I'm going to do if this gets worse." I think I'd forgotten this *could* get any worse. Each day was hell. And the next day would be worse. And on and on.

"Come on," Mom said, her eyes closed, "at least try."

Pa chanted, "Oh-wa-tahgoo-siam."

Kai took his words as his cue and ran to Pa, tugging on his pant leg. "Up," he said. Kai climbed into his lap and pointed at the cars on the street like they always did. Pa held the air in his cheeks and blew it out, making Kai giggle to the point of tears. Pa did it over and over, even though he needed every gasp. After a while Kai settled into his arms and they both smiled peacefully in the chair, looking out the window.

Mom, still kneeling behind the chair, hands extended, opened her eyes and leaned to me whispering, "I told you it worked."

I liked when Mom and Stacie went to Reiki classes because that meant Kai and I could spend alone time with Pa. Someone needed to be around all the time, now, as we worried about another incident occurring, or his BiPAP losing power or shutting down unexpectedly. On one such evening Pa called before I could come over. He apologized, but said he needed the breathing machine—he was running out of air. Kai and I bounded across the backyard and found him in bed. He said he was tired; some days it was too much even to sit upright. I strapped the mask to his face and we turned on the television. Kai climbed next to him and Pa signed words to us to communicate. I'd grown quite deft at reading his signs. The charades took time, and I sometimes struggled to comprehend, but it made each word that much more important. He said he felt like his own dad sitting in a hospital bed. He apologized for making me come over. I told him there wasn't anywhere else I'd rather be. And I meant it. It was nice just to do normal activities like watch TV, despite the circumstances. Kai sat next to my dad, gobbled up snacks, read books, and handed Pa a stuffed dog and a car. Whenever Pa's mask made the suction sound, Kai mimicked it, so Pa started doing it on purpose to make Kai laugh.

We talked about my new Smartboard at school and the stereo I'd just bought. It was a perfect night: three guys watching TV, talking the best they could. It was peace we hadn't had in a while. No tension. No catastrophes. Those moments made me believe this wasn't the end. Or anything at all. Just a moment of normalcy.

The call was all fabric. That's all I could make out—fabric or bristle rubbing against the phone. I ran. Kai and I had been playing in the backyard, and even though he could walk, it would never be fast enough, so I picked up Kai and ran. We recently made the decision not to renew the contract on my dad's smartphone. The buttons were all too small, and, as he stated, "Who the hell am I going to call?" Instead we bought him a pre-paid phone with large buttons—something my grandparents could handle. In that case, if there was an emergency, Pa could just hold down the preloaded numbers and speak to us.

That night Mom and Stacie were again at Reiki, but Pa said he was fine and I should play with Kai outside while the sun was still up. He'd call, he said, if he needed anything. "I'll be fine," he said.

I somehow kept the phone to my ear the entire run with my son under my arm. The whole way the sound on the other end was struggle—the fabric moved more quickly, then something sounded wet.

I set Kai on the floor and burst into his bedroom. The mask was half on, Pa's eyes wide in panic. I pulled on his shoulder, straight up, and he winced. It was too fast. I hurt him. I forgot how much moving hurt. He pointed to his throat. His eyes moved quickly back and forth. They were so pronounced on his face. Then a gurgle. A wheeze. And something cleared. He took a deep breath and pointed to the mask. It had been blowing air the whole time, so I attached it to his face and carefully leaned him back on the bed. He gave me a thumbs up and pointed to his eye. Heart. Then me. I returned the gesture just as slowly and carefully as he did: Eye. Heart. Him.

After he recovered a bit, he requested the mask's removal. It was strange to hear his voice, as we'd all grown used to gestures. Sort of like when Darth Vader removes his mask, it's just not the sound I expected. He explained how he started choking on his spit, but lacked the muscle to clear it. He tried to pull the mask off to call me or clear his throat, but all he could do was panic because he wasn't strong enough to pull the mask off all the way or clear the phlegm. He asked me to bring Kai on the bed. "Robi," Kai said, pointing to the mask resting on Pa's chest. Kai thought Pa looked like a robot when he wore the mask. Kai smiled, leaned into Pa's arm and whispered, "Robi Papa," as I reattached the straps.

When Mom came home I told her. She nodded and stroked his hair lightly, sitting cross-legged on the bed. "I'm going to try the Reiki now," she said. Lately Pa said the Reiki actually calmed him. Mom thought maybe there was something to it. When we lost faith in the gods, we turned to ourselves. Mom and Stacie only had one more class before they were "official." "Then I won't have to leave in the evenings anymore,"

Mom said. "And we can fix you." As Kai and I left the room, Kai slipped one of his Hotwheels cars into his pocket, and I looked back to see Mom by Pa's side, palms extended, trying to heal my dad with all she had.

"I just won't go," Mom said. She didn't look well. Her face was fresh with tears. "I can't leave him again. Last time it was bad—he could have died."

"I'm not going outside tonight," I said. "Kai and I will be right here by Pa's side. I'll call if anything happens."

She ran her hand through her hair, which was slightly unkempt, a few grey hairs out of place. She was losing it. The bathroom wasn't going well anymore—it was hard to transfer him to the toilet, and he even lacked the muscles for basic functions. "He's just all bone," she said between tears. "So much bone." She was exhausted. I could come and go—return to a life of television and a job, distractions she didn't have. "Tonight, before I transferred him to the toilet he said, 'It would just be so nice to stand up and take a shower. That would be nice.' That's all we fucking want. The basics. But God won't even give us that."

I convinced her to go. I didn't know if there would be another night when she could leave—she knew him better than any of us, and she knew his health was spiraling. She knew how to move his body on a board from one seat to another. How to lift him without hurting him. And how to point her palms in his direction to heal him. "Besides," I said, "you need to finish your Jedi training tonight so you can fix him."

"It's all bullshit. It's not doing anything. And tonight he couldn't move his hand. He's losing it all."

"I don't know. He seems to be better when you do it. Calmer at least." It was no longer about healing him. We had to heal her, too.

So they went. Before I put his mask on I asked if there was anything I could do for him. "Start up the zero turn, carry me to the garage, and stick my face to the muffler."

"I wish I could," I said. Kai was cranky that night, refusing to eat any of the food I'd prepared for him. We were in our typical spots for this gathering—Pa in the bed, Kai by his side, and the TV on. That first time was so serene. This night wasn't.

Kai threw a piece of cornbread across the bedroom. I apologized to my dad, scrambling to pick it up.

He shook his head. Told me to relax. He "spoke" with what was left of his hand, since I'd already attached his mask. He flattened it the best he could and moved it across his lap. *Relax.*

I tried to make small talk over the TV—told him the playground company was coming to stake out the playset for Kai this week under the tree, so there's not too much sun. He nodded. I realized he'd never see Kai play on his swing. The trees in their backyard obstructed the view of our house, and he'd never leave his own home again. Not alive.

Kai threw another piece of food.

Pa began choking behind his mask. It started as a slight cough, his chest fluttering, but transgressed into a full-fledged choke. Kai screamed and rocked back and forth. Pa used what he had of his strength to push the mask off his mouth. I reacted, helping him remove it fully. He coughed again, trying to clear the phlegm. But the coughs were silent because without muscle, there is no sound. Kai shrieked again. Minutes of this silent panic. I tried to raise his arms, allow the air to clear it. But each move was pain. He shook his head. Eventually, after enough shifts, it cleared. I asked if he needed anything. He closed his eyes without answering. I gently reattached the mask, but his eyes remained closed.

I took Kai down from the bed and he pointed to my dad. "Not today," I said. "We're going to let Papa rest." My dad licked his lips behind the mask and squeezed his eyes closed tighter. It hurt. It all hurt. His breathing was still off. The coughing returned. But he never opened his eyes. I asked if he wanted the mask off, but he shook his head. Kai played quietly on the ground with a toy car. The gagging continued.

This was it. We'd all been imagining this moment. His skin was pale against his eyelashes. Then the coughing grew more violent. His eyes snapped open. And we repeated. Arms. Pain. Waiting for it to clear. It didn't. Kai scratched the toy car wheels against the ground and my father started to die. In this room. The three of us. "I love you," I said. I had to say it. I didn't know what we were looking at. He closed his eyes again, tighter. Now. Now. Now.

He couldn't even thrash.

I could hear the kitchen door open from the garage. "Mom," I cried. "Mom!"

She came running. I backed away from the chair and she moved his body in a specific twist to the right. It wasn't working. I picked up Kai and took him into the spare room. Mom swore. She swore and swore and said, "No, no, no." Stacie joined me in the room with Kai, and I began to cry. I tried to explain to her what was happening. "This might be it, I tried, but I just don't know."

"Stop it!" Mom screamed. "Stop. It. Clear. Clear goddammit."

And then silence.

I looked at Stacie. We both breathed in sync. Together. Breath. Breath. Kai was silent, too. He stared at us. The house hadn't been that quiet in some time. Ever. Mom began to cry. Stacie and I didn't move. No one dared to flinch.

"Mom," I said in a whisper. "Mom."

"It's okay," she said. "He's okay."

I went to his bedside. She was kneeling next to my dad, who was breathing at regular intervals again, lying peacefully, holding her hand. Rather, she was holding his. Mom was sweaty—still wearing her jacket and shoes. Her hair stuck up and her face was red. With the hand not holding my dad's she had a palm outstretched performing Reiki.

"I need to call the doctor," she said. "I don't know what to do."

Stacie agreed to take Kai home—he didn't need to witness

this—while I watched over Pa when Mom made the call. The house was still so muted. Mom stood in the office across from their bedroom and dialed the phone. Her finger made quiet clicks as she pressed the buttons on the phone, navigating a series of options.

The TV was off now, and Pa rested.

"Daniel Hemery. 9-21-48," Mom said in a hush—not because she was trying to be quiet, but her voice sounded broken, somewhere else. She repeated his name and birthday, "Daniel Hemery. 9-21-48." And again. "Daniel Hemery. 9-21-48."

Her voice was too quiet to make out every word, but I caught bits of, "How to clear," "could have died," and "yes, I'll hold."

"Daniel Hemery. 9-21-48." How many times did she have to say it? To identify him. Verify him. She was on the phone for over forty minutes. She hung up the receiver gently. Sighed a breath that filled the room, and came back to her bedroom.

"I don't understand it. I don't fucking understand how they can just abandon us like this." She said it took a half-hour to get to a doctor, "And when I finally reached him, you know what he said? He said, 'I've never treated Daniel, so I can't give you any advice.' I said you can't tell me how to clear the throat of an ALS patient and he said no. He said no." I held her hand. "They told me to take him to the ER if it's not clearing and I asked exactly how I was to transport him, and they said to call an ambulance." She lowered her voice. "You know how badly those bumps would hurt him?" She finally pulled off her jacket. "Fucking worthless."

"Why couldn't the doctor tell you what to do?" I asked.

"He said because it wasn't his patient and Pa's doctor was on vacation. And then he asked why we haven't been in for a visit lately to check his numbers." She began to cry.

The mask began to suction. And he began to choke.

"No, no, no!" she said. She pulled his body again upright. The mask fell off.

"Come on, Hemery," Pa screamed as loudly as he could between gasps. "Take care of that fucking mask." It wasn't the gagging this time, but the mask wasn't sealing properly, choking him behind the plastic. Mom was working meticulously through the tears that fell all over the mask and my dad. He gasped harder.

"Faster," he said. "Fucking faster."

"I'm goddamn trying!"

"Just let me die. Just let me die," Pa said.

She secured the mask and his eyes immediately relaxed. She leaned on the bed. She was done. Her job was to keep alive a dying man who wanted to go. Lately they had these moments of screaming and shouting, my dad frustrated not by my mom, but by it all. They went after each other because that's what they had. Each other. Mom had rearranged the entire bedroom to fit a wheelchair he began using. She could get him from the chair in the living room to the wheelchair because they were on the same level, but the bed was higher. It was a new one that Mom bought that could contour and adjust to the curve of my dad's back. But it filled the room, and she didn't have the strength to lift his dead weight. The first time she tried, she called in a panic for me to help him. Just this once. She told me repeatedly that this wasn't my job, that she'd figure it out for next time. The problem was the 90-degree angle of the wheelchair without the BiPAP—he couldn't breathe. So those seconds in transfer were like drowning. And the longer it took, the more panicked he became. The angrier he grew. That day when I came over, once I pulled his body to the bed, he snapped at Mom, and said, "I can't goddamn breathe in that chair. I fucking need you to be ready when I am." Mom fell to the floor without words, anguish. Both were breathless.

ALS is not Stephen Hawking—technology at the ready. It was two breathless soul mates in a small living room with barely the space for a wheelchair. A woman who wanted so desperately to keep her husband breathing that she sacrificed it all. Every hour. Every moment. And no help from the medical community because orphan diseases are just that, orphans. They lack the glitz and universality of other diseases. They are nearly forgotten.

After the rough transfer Mom stood up from the couch and stormed to the basement and then returned. She screamed, "People think we have for fucking ever to figure out this wheelchair situation. We don't have forever. We no longer have forever." The last time Pa's therapist called to see if she could put him in the car and drive him to an appointment (house calls were never an option), she spoke with Pa on the phone to ensure he wasn't suicidal again. She asked him if he ever thought about killing himself. Pa said, "Every hour of every day." The therapist laughed off the comment, but Pa assured her he wasn't joking. Pa explained that every day is the "same damn thing. The same damn chair every day." The therapist told him he "needed to make memories. We don't leave much else behind." She encouraged my dad to "get out of the house" and see our new playset. When Mom took the phone to ask how to move him and get him out of the house, the therapist swore she'd send a specialist to look into the transfer situation. A new chair. All sorts of potentials. Despite Mom's frequent calls to her office at the hospital, no one ever came.

It was the ALS Association who continued to step up to equip Mom with anything she needed. Since Pa's data wasn't available to the hospital, he wasn't interesting to them anymore.

As for Mom, her desperation was immense, but we didn't know what else to do. We made her meals, so she didn't have to always cook and watch after Pa. I offered her nights off, but she wouldn't have it. She never left in the evening, except to train in Reiki. He was better in the morning because he had more strength, so she'd sneak out for a few minutes, but never for an extended period of time. And she never asked anyone for anything—except the simple request of a doctor on how to clear the throat of her partner of forty years. How to keep him alive a little longer.

That night, when we nearly lost my dad to his own spit, she looked broken in every sense of the word. She told me to go. That there was nothing else to be done. We'd all look at this again tomorrow, she said.

"What are you going to do?" I asked.

"Just stay here," she said. "There's nothing else to do, but stay right here." She stood up, kissed me on the head, and pulled my sweatshirt hood up for me. I leaned over the bed and kissed my dad. All bones. Something that once was. She kneeled back by the bedside and outstretched her palms toward him. I let myself out, locking the kitchen door behind me. It was raining and dark, the mud seeping into my shoes as I made the journey home.

Years prior my dad told me to write a eulogy for my grandfather when he had a stroke, after he began to piss himself in his home, unable to stand on his own, right before we put him in a nursing home. "It will be soon," Pa told me. It wasn't. He was still alive, nearly five years later. And he would now outlive my father. I never wrote the eulogy like my dad asked—it seemed dark to anticipate death. But now, I began to think of my father's night, when we would stand before a room of people and speak of my dad's kindness. Because in his bedroom, that night was a preview. It would surely end like this. She would have to say his name again someday. His birthdate. Prove his existence. And it would be the end.

I missed him already.

46. Broken

When I was in my twenties, our seventy-something-pound German Shepherd mix, Cherry, snapped a rabbit's back and left it for dead one winter night in our backyard. This wasn't the first time—she'd long had the reputation of killing rabbits, opossums, mice, squirrels and anything else with fur in our backyard. I'd always been squeamish about death. My dad would kindly trudge across the backyard to pick up whatever carnage Cherry left. "What are you going to do when I'm gone?" he asked me once.

"Have a yard full of dead things," I answered.

Aside from the family of opossums, which he picked up by their tails, he always wrapped a garbage bag around his hand and picked up the animals. "Can't you feel them through the bag?" I asked.

"Well, yeah," he said. "But what's the big deal? It's dead."

I first spotted the rabbit through the kitchen window. Its body moved unnaturally, twisting how a body shouldn't, alone in the backyard. It was dark, so only the deck lights illuminated the white blur. When I called my dad to tell him, he sighed and hung up the phone. I could see him walking through the yard with a garbage bag hanging out of his jeans pocket. He knelt next to the rabbit and shook his head. The bag still dangling, he reached out, bare handed, and picked up the creature.

"Pa," I shouted from the deck. "Pa, what are you going to do?" I worried he'd take care of it like the mouse that we caught years before, the trap slicing its head, but not killing it. He gathered him in a small box and carried him to the garage, crushing him with a brick. "Pa!"

He didn't respond. Maybe I didn't want to know.

I called Mom and asked what he was doing, but she said she hadn't a clue. That he'd been in the garage for an hour or more. "Should you check on him?" I asked.

"I don't even want to know what he's doing," she said, having seen him behead a mole with a shovel that was digging up his garden.

It wasn't until the next morning when I called that I heard what he'd done. There was no shovel or brick. Instead, he nestled the rabbit into the warmth of his jacket. "The poor little thing was having a rough time," he said. "So I just kept him warm. I could see in his eyes he wasn't going to make it through the night, so I figured I might as well make his last few hours comfortable." So he stayed that way, in the garage, with a white rabbit nuzzled into his arms like a newborn, for hours, until it was gone and he blew out his last breaths of warm steam in the cold winter's night.

47. Fighting Monsters

Stacie and I discussed it a lot. We had to. Stacie was unfortunate enough to lose both of her parents before she was twenty-seven. She'd seen them both die in front of her—cancer, a few years apart. One day we were saying how unfair this was for Pa. "There's no guarantees," she said. "I think we expect *the* story—the birth, the jobs, the kids, retiring, and passing in our loved one's arms at ninety. That's the narrative we've been told our whole lives. But there are no guarantees."

"So why do we do it? Why do we keep going every day?" I asked.

"Because we must believe in *it*. That *it's* worth it. I mean, we had a kid so we must believe in a future. Death is just an unfortunate side effect."

There was a noise in the adjacent room. I paused to hear if Kai was awake—he'd been napping quietly. It was only the house shifting.

"But this all just sucks. This disease is the worst," Stacie said. "It shouldn't be surprising that mankind does horrible things to each other like genocide or whatever—because just look at the cruelty of nature—like that show last night." We'd been watching a PBS special on falcons. In the one scene the falcon hides itself in the brightness of the sun and then silently drops to the earth to tear a rabbit into ribbons. "Nature is awful. And this, this rotten cruel disease, well, it seems just as bad as anything man could create. We are a product of our world."

"I think the worst part," I said, changing direction a bit, "is seeing him like that. This man that was larger than life, the most physically gifted person I know, well, to see him frail and falling apart. It's just not right. I'll never forget the first time I knew how strong he was, and it was a little thing, but in junior high there was this group of boys that would pick on me. Relentlessly. Well, my folks and I always went grocery shopping on Friday nights—we'd get dinner at Taco Bell or whatever, we'd go grocery shop, and then they'd buy me frozen yogurt. We did this even when the other kids were probably not hanging out with their parents, but, I don't know, I still liked just being with them. They made more sense than kids my age. Anyhow, so this one time we pulled into the frozen yogurt shop parking lot and there they all were—Jeff and Jimmy and all these kids that made my life hell. They were all sitting on BMX bikes in the parking lot, smoking. Fourteen years old and smoking. And I said to Pa, 'Hey, we probably shouldn't go here, because there are some bad kids who want to hurt me here.' And do you know what he said? He just looked at me and said, 'I've never been afraid.' But I kept going and tried to explain how big they were and how the one had huge muscles. But he just said, 'Kiddo, I could take on every one of them at once. And win. Big.' Up to that point I'd never really thought about it. I mean, sure, he was an adult, but those kids seemed huge to me back then. But I'll never forget that moment because I knew he would always have my back and he was stronger than whatever my biggest problem was. And he lived his whole life that way, protecting me from whatever the monsters were in my closet. Except he can't fight this one off."

We were sitting at the tiled-kitchen table and Stacie traced the lines of grout with her finger. "But he's still that, even now," she said.

"How can you say that? He can't even move his body. He's gone. Broken."

"Look at him, Mike. Seriously. Your dad is a bad motherfucker. Even now he's a bad motherfucker. He's taking this on, not to beat it, he knows he can't, but he's not going to let anyone let him live past a certain point. He won't be trached. He won't take a feeding tube. He's going to go down his way. He's the strongest man I've ever met in my life. Even unable to move or sometimes breathe, he's still taking care of things. One bad motherfucker."

I nodded. She was right. It was the most helpful thing anyone had said to me since he was diagnosed. I hummed the chorus of the famous Neil Young song: "It's better to burn out, than to fade away."

Stacie continued. She's not usually a talker—she listens and gives advice, but she won't go on and on. But today she seemed to find it necessary, probably because she knew I needed it. "Think about yesterday—identity theft and the 'Dan in the Can' conversations."

The previous day we were visiting, and Mom and Pa were talking about identity theft because Pa had been watching a lot of television and noticed the commercials for protecting yourself against someone taking your identity. "Can you imagine the surprise on those bastards' faces if they stole my identity. They'd think they were getting some cash, and all they'd get is entombment. Surprise!"

He started laughing, which made Kai begin to laugh and chant, "Robi Papa, Robi Papa."

Pa nodded and said, "Right, kiddo? You get it."

The conversation then moved to what to do with his ashes when he'd gone. He brought it up. Pa said to take the ashes to France and dump them over the cliffs in Fécamp, his hometown, into the ocean. He said he'd like to be there. He grew up on those cliffs and always wondered what it would be like to fall from the cliffs into the ocean. Stacie latched onto the practical and said we wouldn't know how to communicate in French without him. On our last major vacation together we all went to Fécamp, where my dad came alive with the glint of a child, showing us the statue he and his buddies spray painted—a controversy not even Grandma knew about. And the place where his swimming "instructor" threw him into the ocean and told him to move all his limbs or he'd sink to the bottom. It was a great trip because he seamlessly slipped back into being French.

"Here's what I'll do," he said. It was early in the day so his voice was strong. "I'll write down…"

Mom interrupted him, "Using your good arm?" He smiled.

"Shut up. Anyhow, I'll write some key translations on the urn so you can just carry me around talking to people. Just pack me in your luggage. 'Dan in a Can.'" We all laughed ourselves silly, even Kai.

"Even that," Stacie now said at the kitchen table. "Think about it. He's looking down the barrel of death. Straight in the goddamn eye, and he's laughing the entire time. He's still that guy from your youth. Your father is one bad motherfucker."

She was young — maybe in her mid-to-late twenties. Her short, spikey hair was blond in the moonlight of the driveway, and even brighter as she approached the fluorescent garage lighting. She carried two bags — a large duffle with a red cross on it and a laptop bag. As she walked up the drive I wasn't sure who should speak first, what was the protocol in these situations. I nodded as her shoes scraped across the concrete, more to confirm she'd made it to the right place, as that would be an awkward slip of an address.

She smiled, stopping in the garage to adjust the straps of the bags. "How are you?" she said.

I said hello. I didn't see how it was possible to answer her question.

"Are we ready to do this?" she asked, her vocal pitch high and energetic. She smacked the gum in her mouth and began chomping down hard.

Taken aback by her comment, which didn't seem to match the moment, didn't match the gravity of the room a few steps from where we stood, I felt the need to clarify. "My dad is in there." I pointed through the drywall of the garage. "He wants his mask off. To die." I needed to say it, because her words made it sound like we were going for a walk or to hem his pants.

"This is my first time doing one of these," she said. *One of these.* "But it should be fine." *Should.*

I stared at her. "You're from hospice?" I asked. This didn't make sense, the flip manner in which she spoke. She nodded and clicked her gum. I breathed in the cold air. "We spoke with the doctor and the plan is to give him enough morphine so that he is relaxed and then remove the mask. We've already given him our doses that we had left."

"Sounds like a plan," she said, smiling. My face must have given myself away, as she quickly countered with, "I'm so sorry about your mom—dad, I mean." I blinked. She looked toward the door. "Should we go in? It's nippy out here tonight." I blinked again.

I led her into the kitchen, where Mom was waiting. Mom's face was worn. Her hair was grayer, her spirit tired. I left the two to speak in the kitchen and went to be with my dad.

He called me over. His mask was on, but he nodded his head, motioning for me to remove it. I did. It beeped its warning.

"Kiddo. Do me a favor," he said.

"Anything."

He breathed hard. "I need to go tonight. Don't let them fuck this up." He smiled, gasping for breath.

I smiled back while I reattached the mask. Kissing him on the head I said, "They're in the business of dying—it'll be fine."

48. Where We Were

Each change was jarring. But to reflect upon what was now normal was equally as unnerving. Kai only knew Robi Papa—his earlier memories of my dad unplugged and still able to walk were replaced by a man stationary in a chair. In the beginning of the disease, when Pa could still walk, Kai would giggle at his odd pacing. As it progressed, he knew the cue when Mom moved to my dad to conduct something more serious—a seat transfer with a lift strap or trying to clear dinner from the throat. He understood he must move, usually backing his little body against mine to remain out of the way.

But my dad still watched out for Kai the best he could. After I explained to my dad an incident at library story time where a mother indifferently scolded Kai when he accidentally fell and hit his head on her shoe, Pa told me we should go back and teach Kai the word "bitch."

But Kai only knew my dad's failing shell. Pa once said during a visit, "The body instinctively fights to survive—another design flaw of us mammals." But Kai didn't comprehend any of that darkness, so when Mom finished with her procedures, he'd charge my dad, asking to watch train videos on his laptop. He'd rest on my dad's lap until his breathing waned, and I'd remove him to keep Pa alive. He knew that version. Pa said he and his grandson understood each other because they both drank out of sippy cups, otherwise unsteady hands would spill their drinks. Kai was gentler with my dad than any of us, like he instinctively knew. One day he tottered over to my dad and offered him a slug of his sippy cup, said, "Hugs," and embraced his knee. Then Kai walked over to my mom and head butted her.

Most of the changes were for the worse, except for the BiPAP nose piece the ALS Association delivered to Mom. The device fitted into the BiPAP tube, but instead of covering his entire mouth, it only went into his nose, allowing him to speak while simultaneously receiving ample amounts of air. At first his voice was full of tenor and vibrated when he spoke. Plus, if he opened his mouth and didn't regulate his nose, air whooshed out of his mouth from the nose piece. Kai laughed and said he "sounded funny." But with some practice he was able to be there again, part of the room. There was no more pantomiming or distance. He was part of life again. So we talked and laughed freely, like old times. While drinking a glass of wine in my parents' living room, Stacie said, "This wine is making my muscles relax."

Although he couldn't drink wine anymore—it stuck in his throat—my dad grinned and said, "Mine, too."

For some reason that simple change lifted all of our spirits. Before my dad was half gone, but now he was back in it, and that small piece of plastic actually provided some more false hope that things weren't as dismal as they seemed. Pa and I talked about everything. When he ran out of stories I told him about the drum set I was going to buy. During college, I'd sold the original one he and I bought when I was fourteen. We snuck out when Mom was running errands and returned with a massive seven-piece sparkling red Tama Superstar kit with cymbals and hi-hats, the works. I had the itch again and told him what I was going to buy, and even brought over one of the toms after I made the purchase. We talked a lot about the beach and "our" park in Rocky River, where we could watch a day slip away by staring at the boats lazily sailing by and the children building castles in the sand.

When I decided to have my driveway replaced I brought over Mr.

Spanulo, the son of the laborer who redid my dad's driveway years before. He spoke to my dad through the living room window. "You're a legend in our shop," Spanulo said.

"Why?" my dad asked.

"You're the guy who dug your foundation with a shovel—a fucking shovel!"

It was true. When the foundation of my dad's house began to crack and buckle, he'd spend every night after work meticulously digging down ten feet, nearly the entire perimeter of his home. The job took all summer, but he did it and replaced all the dirt with stone for better drainage.

"Man, it's cool to finally meet you," Spanulo said. "My dad always talked about this guy, this beast, who did it with a shovel!"

My dad smiled.

But the nose piece was witchery. Because despite his stick-frame, for a moment, when he spoke and when people spoke about him, it was easy to forget. After months of silence because of the mask, we all thought maybe he was getting better. His skin looked better. He could laugh without being stifled. He was that man who dug his foundation out with a shovel, and even if only for a moment, I believed maybe he would be able to do that again.

A few days after Spanulo's visit I called my parents to check on things. No one answered. Someone always answered. I called again. Answering machine. I told Stacie I'd be right back—that I wanted to check on my folks.

When I got there Mom was in the kitchen, red-faced and throwing pans into the cupboard.

"Everything okay?" I asked, removing my shoes.

"No, Mike, everything is not okay," she said.

"What's going on?"

"Nothing. Nothing is going on. It's all just falling to shit."

"Well, what happened?"

"Mike, just drop it, will you?" She threw the towel that was on her shoulder into the kitchen sink. "I don't want to fucking rehash it all. Just drop it." She pushed me aside, threw open the basement door and stomped down the stairs.

ALS is dying in a slow motion car wreck, seeing the other vehicle slowly approach out of control. It works its way from the foot, to ankle, to shin for months, the knee, stomach, compression of the chest, slowly crushing you in your own rigging. It wears away at your family structure, testing everyone's nerves, driving you insane as you lose the most important person in your life. It makes you furious, raging—it'd been eight months since my dad had left the house. Stir crazy, tired, in pain. "Enough," Mom said. She surrendered. Her research for a cure was coming to an end. She was stretched too far. "Enough."

I went to the living room to see what had happened. Apparently Mom was giving him a bath in his chair, but insisted on washing his face. He couldn't hold his head up and was cold, so he started gasping and turning purple. All she wanted for her husband was to wash his face, but the disease won't allow its victims any luxuries. So he gasped. And he said she looked horrified and cried and apologized and kept repeating, "You looked dead. Your skin, the way you looked, you looked dead."

Despite the freedom and hope that new nose piece gave us, we all knew. And Mom unfortunately had the preview of what happens when the body changes quickly and the life drains. This moment brought us back. There wasn't much "okay" left. Pa said he wished he could do more, but he felt like she was cracking, that maybe it was all too much.

She came loudly back up the stairs, and Pa quickly changed the topic to the Google Earth site he'd been looking at. Mom stormed by with her blue laundry baskets. "What are you two jerks talking about?" Mom asked. She sighed and continued on to the bedroom.

"Just looking at the planet," Pa answered. "Dropping pinpoints where we are and where we were."

49. Dreaming Without Him

A pedophile was rushing through our house looking for Kai. I broke a beer bottle and chased him through the streets to a prison cell. But then the jail cell became a Mexican fort with stucco walls and dust-covered accoutrements. I asked a man near the entrance for the ambassador and in walked a man in full regalia—a multi-colored poncho and a hat that looked a bit like a donkey—who called himself Ricky Pratt. We fought with knives for a while until he declared me the winner. I quickly turned and left the fort to find a beautiful blond woman with ample cleavage spilling from a low-cut shirt sitting atop a llama. She was wearing cutoff jean shorts, with her shirt tied well above the navel. I leapt in front of her on the llama and reached back to smack the blonde's butt, shouting, "Hi-Ya!"

She whispered, "My father is watching."

I answered, "I know."

And we, rather slowly, trotted away on the back of the llama.

I woke up relieved. It was the first dream in a while without disease or decay. The first in a while with a happy ending, albeit slow.

50. Paths

He called me over because his drains were all gurgling. From his chair he could hear the sputtering in the kitchen and bathroom. "Sounds like a sewage plant in here," he said. I grabbed Kai and trudged to my parents' house. It was the last day of my summer break. The air was still warm, but the breeze suggested cooler days ahead. On my way over I saw the city water company truck outside his house. I waved down a worker, and he explained they were blowing air in the lines—routine maintenance.

"Damn city," Pa said when I relayed the message. "Always messing with something."

"You look like hell," I said.

Pa laughed; the air from the nose piece blew out his mouth. "Why thank you." Kai ran to the toy box in the corner of the room and pulled out some cars.

"Seriously, you look like you've been hit by a truck. What happened?"

"I wish I'd be hit by a truck." The drain gurgled. "It's just been a bad week. Last night I fell during the transfer into bed. And the bathroom thing is still hell." The muscle loss affected every moment, and bowel movements could take hours. "I just feel bad for your mom." He began to cry. I hadn't seen him cry much in these two years; he usually held it together. He never felt sorry for himself, but his empathy was always for Mom. And things were getting worse. The transfers from the bed to the toilet were physically and emotionally draining for both of them.

Their fights were loud. I called two nights before and Mom answered the phone with no *hello*, but, "It's all goddamn fucking shit. It's all falling apart over here." And an hour later she was at our back door hugging Stacie and me, telling us how much she loved us. We didn't blame her. We just respected her strength. I'd seen her land the transfers time and time again. I'd also witnessed the few misses. Pa told me once to stick around to see how great Mom did, but unfortunately something skidded and missed. Before anyone knew it, Pa was screaming, "I swear to God…" and Mom retorted with "Fucking goddamn!" She'd never let me help because she said, "It wasn't my burden" and "What if you're not here." Pa called later that night to tell me what a solid transfer into bed Mom gave him. Despite the explosions, the wounds healed themselves almost instantly.

Now he sat crying in gasps, because he lacked the strength to even mourn properly. Silent cries and wet eyes. "It's all falling apart, but not fast enough. I wish I would have at least tried to kill myself when I could still move—at least tried letting that car run long enough, put my face right into that tailpipe. Now I don't know what to do."

I said, "But at least you had two more years with Mom, us and Kai."

"I should be playing cars with him. Right now. Next year. When he's ten. I loved playing cars with you and I'd love playing with him. But I can't. Anyways, Kai won't remember me." I joined him with tears. They say memories start sticking at three. My earliest memory was movement, my dad walking me through the house at night, the floorboards creaking as he tried to soothe me to sleep. Then the warmth of my dad's hair—probably being carried on his back, the sun baking his hair with heat. Surely Kai would remember the window, the crook of my dad's arm, or the sound of the breathing machine. But my dad was right, and I worried how much time would pass before our little one would stop saying "Papa."

"You know that movie *The Suicide Tourist*," Pa began, his tears now dry. He spoke about the film all the time. "The U.S. should allow it—it's right, you know? I think if anyone who makes laws could see me, they'd see that it's the right thing to do. Just let people die. The whole thing was so peaceful. He just clicked this timer to cut off the air. And he went to sleep. The guy looked just like me." Pa breathed. "And his wife was with him and she was okay with it."

I nodded, unsure of what to say.

"Would you do that?" I asked.

"Yes." The quickest and strongest he'd sounded in months. Without hesitation. He repeated himself. "Yes. I'm a shell. This isn't living."

Kai looked up. He'd been playing so intently on the ground, seemingly ignoring all that we'd been saying.

"Papa?" Kai said.

"Yes, Kai?"

"Papa?"

"Yes?"

"Funny." Kai laughed. So did Pa. Kai put his head on my dad's leg, said, "Funny" again, and then returned to his cars, running them up and down the carpet, imaginary streets leading to somewhere where life-sustaining masks were still funny.

51. Little Surprises (Bedsores are Fun)

"It took forty years, but I finally convinced your father to sleep naked," Mom declared to us.

"Too much information," I said, waving my hands at Mom. We'd just stopped over to drop off dinner and check on things when Mom informed us of the news. Pa was chuckling in the living room.

"Those bedsores," Mom explained, "are giving your father hell. They've been bleeding, but when I dress them, his clothes bunch up and the wrinkles hurt him. So, last night he slept in the buff." She grinned. "But then we had an unexpected moment at midnight." The BiPAP started screaming in the living room, as Pa was laughing too hard, disturbing the airflow. "Don't die out there," Mom shouted, while putting the lasagna into the fridge.

"Anyhow," she continued. "You know that new bed we bought for him?" I nodded. It was a thousand-dollar bed that could lift at multiple points and had a massage/vibrate feature. "Well, in the middle of the night the thing starts shaking us to pieces. It was the damnedest thing. Woke us both up. We had no idea what was going on. Turns out—I always put the remote for the bed on Pa's belly so he can adjust it in the middle of the night if the angle of the bed is giving him pain. Well, last night, without clothes..." Mom nodded her head like we should be able to fill in the rest.

"What?" I asked.

"You know."

"I don't know."

The BiPAP screamed.

Stacie started snickering.

"His 'stuff' accidentally hit the vibrate button in the middle of the night. Quite the way to wake up, let me tell you."

Stacie and I let out a series of loud "Ohmygawds" and "OhJeezes." Pa laughed and laughed from the other room, the BiPAP singing along with him.

"I guess that will be the last time he sleeps that way," Stacie said.

Mom smirked and said, "Oh, I don't know about that."

52. Locked In

She needed to get out. Stacie and I (with Kai and the dog in tow) knocked on my parents' front door, asking Mom to go for a walk around the neighborhood with us. She hesitated to leave my dad alone. He now required the BiPAP all day and needed the air to survive. But he pointed to the cell phone on the table and made a motion with his hands. "Go, go," he mouthed through the window.

"It'd be good to get out for a bit," I said. She conceded, switched his mask to the nose piece in case he needed to call, locked the front door and exited out of the garage.

The early October air was just turning, the light crispness cutting through our jackets. Autumn has the best light, making its subjects look more alive right before they burn out into winter. Mom seemed relaxed—able just to talk without worrying if the mask was blowing its seal or stressing over if she should be investigating a new trial for my dad. The last one she suggested turned into an evening discussion with us all—whether transporting my dad to Johns Hopkins was worth it. Despite my dad's wishes to be left alone to die, Mom put his name on the waiting list because they were only taking fifteen ALS patients. She was later informed that he didn't make the cut. As it turned out, the trial was a failure.

"The pictures are fun, at least," Mom said. Every evening she and my dad had been scanning all of their old slides into the computer to digitize their past, preserving it in whatever way they could. "We looked so young back then. And your father was so handsome. He's such a good looking man." Her voice was of course tinged with sadness, but there was something joyous in it, too. "It's just a good thing for us to do. He sits in the wheelchair with the BiPAP for as long as his back will allow, and we scan and hold hands and cry. But it's nice. It is. Sort of feels like a nice way to say goodbye to each and every moment we've had together."

We didn't have much alone time with Mom anymore, so even the brief fifteen-minute walk around the neighborhood was satisfying, a reprieve during which everyone could pretend like this was okay and that the fall air was something to be celebrated. As we rounded the corner to their house, Pa waved from the front window, and Mom opened the garage door and turned the handle of the inside door. "Love you," I said, waving from the driveway.

"Wait," she cried, her voice shrill.

I turned to witness her twisting the handle back and forth, pushing her weight at the door. "Did you lock this?" she yelled.

"I didn't even leave with you," I said, all of us returning to the garage.

She tried her key in the deadbolt, but that wasn't the problem. The top lock, the one none of us have ever had a key to had somehow dropped into the lock position.

"Goddammit," she cried, pushing more forcefully on the door.

I called Pa immediately. "How the hell?" he asked.

"I don't know, but what I do know is we can't get in." And he had no way of standing to let us in.

Mom grew more desperate, her eyes filled with tears. "What if the machine fails or the power goes off and I can't…fucking…get in there." She pushed, but the lock did what the lock was designed to do. In that moment we all realized just how vulnerable my father's life was, susceptible to everything from power outages to botched transfers from his seat to a failed lock on a door. He sat in his chair at the front window, locked in, twice, his body and now his home.

"Vise grips," he whispered. "Get my vise grips from the toolbox."

He walked me through the process. I crushed the handle, ripping it from its casing, then carefully used the needle-nose pliers to pull out a small piece of metal that was keeping the lock in place. Mom asked if I knew what I was doing. I said no, but listened to my dad carefully walk me through the directions. He couldn't see the handle, but he could—a testament to his vast knowledge of all things. The entire handle gave way to a gaping hole. "Push it open and you're done," he said on the phone, hanging up without saying goodbye.

Mom rushed past me to check on my dad. Stacie and Kai went home since everything was secure, and I entered the living room carrying the mangled handle and said, "Victory."

"Go change it with another one," Pa said.

It was late and I was tired. The sun had already set, and I hadn't eaten dinner.

"I don't care if you're tired. Go fix it," he said.

"I'm doing my best, Pa. I'm sorry I'm not you. I'll just tape up the hole for tonight and fix it tomorrow."

"I don't care if you're tired. Go. Fix. It."

It wasn't enough that he worked through me, but I had to finish it, like he would. There was no *tired* in my dad's vocabulary. You finished things. Mom told me not to worry about it, that she'd run up to the store and get a replacement. I said I'd stay, but she insisted it wasn't my worry.

When I called later that evening, she said Pa calmed down. He walked her through the steps to replace the handle and they were in the office scanning pictures. Simultaneously, when I said something about the door, the two broke into laughter. "Sorry," she said, after quieting down. "These pictures are so funny. There is one of us camping and your father's hair is so long. He's making this funny face and I'm smiling. That was a good trip."

"Everything's okay, then?"

"Everything is fine."

53. Pa Said

“The box is getting smaller.”

54. Pause

Mom called to tell me to look at the rainbow in the southern sky. Standing on my front step, my bare feet cold against the concrete, I couldn't quite take it all in. It was bright—most times rainbow colors are faded, like an afterthought of color, but this one was different. I'd been so enraptured with the sky, I lost awareness of my surroundings, but was brought back when I heard the flick of a lighter. Don, the man who lived across the street with his girlfriend and her kid, flicked his lighter, holding it to the end of his cigarette. He'd lost his mom a few years back and now lived in her house across the street. He stared up at the rainbow, too, taking a long drag from his cigarette. He scratched his shirtless chest and flicked ashes to the ground. I looked back up, and the rainbow now began to fade somewhat. *I'll be like Don, soon*, I thought. A parent gone. Partially orphaned. The other woman across the street had come out of her house, probably to see what we were doing, and she now looked up at the rainbow, too. The whole neighborhood showed up for a bit of color in the sky. Just then a light mist of rain began to fall—that early autumn rain when nothing is quite official, yet. "That's something," she shouted across the street to Don, pointing to the rainbow. Don nodded and took another drag of his cigarette. "Yeah," she repeated, "that's something."

55. Shadows at Night

He gently rocked my shoulder, then whispered my name. It was dark, save for a blurry light dampened by the van's tinted sunroof. "Mikers, can you wake up?" I blinked away the darkness, focused on my dad kneeling inside our full-sized green van, his sleeping bag rolled away from me. Mom stirred in her bag on the other side, but did not wake up.

I was eight, and this was the final day at Salt Fork. Each year my dad would use his limited vacation days from his job at the printing press so we could camp, sleeping in the van at night and hiking trails during the day. Each morning Mom and Pa would wake up well before me. Mom cooked bacon and pancakes on the small propane griddle right outside the van. Pa kept her company, sipping coffee from a blue, speckled tin mug. Sometimes I'd brave the morning frost for breakfast on a picnic bench and sometimes the three of us would remain folded into each other in the van, until I licked the remaining syrup that clung to my plate, my parents' coffee steaming the windows.

That night my dad wiped the condensation from the side window of the van, squinted at something in the distance, and looked back toward me. I used my elbow to prop my body up, working my way to my dad while still cocooned in my bag. In one motion he pulled me by the arm and tucked me under his wing.

"What's wrong?" I whispered.

"Nothing is wrong," he said. "I wanted you to see something." He moved his face close to mine, so we'd see like one. He raised his finger between our faces and pointed. I followed the path from his knuckle to fingernail to van window to the overhead light on a pole that illuminated our camp spot.

"The light?" I asked.

I could feel his head nod, still pressed against my face. "Just watch."

And in that moment the light flickered. Not because of wavering current, but something passed between the light and us. And again. Then many shadows moved between us, dark objects interrupting the light.

"What is it?" I asked.

I could feel my dad smile in the pause, his cheeks raising. He whispered, "Bats."

I must have gasped or whimpered because Mom woke in a fit, shouting *whatisits* and *iseverythingokays*. I couldn't check on her because I'd planted myself against my father's side, arms holding on tightly. Swarms of blackness flitted outside our van.

"Are we going to be okay?" I asked. Mom now joined us at the window, muttering how we scared the "bajeezus" out of her.

"Of course we're okay," Pa said. "They're just bats." All I knew of bats were from my comic books—animals that when not transforming into sharp-toothed upright figures still craved human blood. Pa messed up my hair and kissed the top of my head. "It's really amazing to see this many and so close."

As the swarm shifted, stray bats would careen toward our van, just barely missing the windows.

I lessened my grip of my father, but remained under his arm. Mom rested her head on mine. None of us spoke. Except for our breathing, all I could hear were the fluttering of hundreds of bat wings. A clamor of stretching skin.

"How do they know where they are going? It seems like that many would be running into each other," I said.

"They have a sense we don't have," Pa said. "Echolocation—something like radar."

"I have radar," I said.

"Oh yeah?"

I slipped out of my sleeping bag and crawled to the other side of the van, turning my back to my folks. "I know you're in the van and I'm not even looking."

Just then my dad leaned across the van and began tickling my sides. I melted into a giggling, kicking mess on the floor as I tried to fend him off. "Where was your radar then?" my dad asked, laughing while he continued to poke the sides of my belly.

Mom hushed us, saying we were going to scare away the bats. My dad returned to the window next to Mom, but I remained on my back, staring up at the skylight. The light in the van strobed as the bats continued to swarm. The closer bats drew deep shadows up the van's walls, perfectly drawn shadow puppets with wings and heads and feet.

After investigating the other windows I returned to the position between my folks—my dad had already discovered the best spot for the show. It was there that we carried on for the remainder of the night. Pa said maybe he'd go outside at one point to see if they'd run into him. But Mom convinced him to just stay there with us. Like fireworks we pointed and *ooo'd* and *ahhh'd* when a particularly striking maneuver occurred or when their tiny feet grazed the window. Mom poured coffee for Pa and herself from a thermos. He asked if I wanted a sip, but I said no, that I just wanted to watch the bats.

And we did, until I grew drowsy, hypnotized by the frantic organization, the patterns of black. I fought the nighttime, but woke the next morning still by the window, covered in a sleeping bag, bacon crackling outside the open sliding door. I hurried to the window, squinted into condensation and the morning sun to see if any bats remained, some stragglers who still twirled about.

"They're gone," my dad said as he crawled back into the van with a plate of food for me.

"So it wasn't a dream?" I asked. "It was real?"

My dad nodded, helping Mom back into the van with the other plates of food. "Yeah," he said, pressing his finger against the moisture on the window. He traced out a head, two wings, and feet. "It was real." We chattered about the previous night, interrupting each other's stories of near misses and flight patterns. I flapped my arms and Pa poked my side, asking why I didn't use my radar.

While Mom and Pa stacked the plates and took them outside to be washed I looked back out the window. The bat my dad had drawn was nearly gone, the water droplets streaked down the window as the sun filled the van.

56. Six Minutes

"What do you mean, six minutes?" I asked, sitting on the floor, perched against my bass drum. I hadn't heard Stacie or Kai come down the stairs. A few of my writer friends and I started a cover band—redoing songs our own way, Beatles songs with a reggae soul, Sublime, and Pearl Jam. Stacie would take Kai out for trips when we'd practice in the basement because we were loud (obnoxious). She said I was having a mid-life crisis. I probably was—coping with the first real stress in my life by engaging in these moments of irresponsibility, but it worked. Whatever the reason, we played music, and we were good. For a little bit, when I sat behind that kit, life felt whole again. I'd record some of the songs for my dad, playing them when I'd visit. He'd shake his head and laugh. It must have been hard—his own hands gone so he could no longer pick up his new guitar and play. He told me the day before that he'd had a dream that he could play again, the chords linking in his dream. "Then I woke up." He said that was the hardest part. "When I dream it's okay, I can move again, but then I wake up. I always wake up."

Our bass player had just flaked out and bailed on the practice after only being there for ten minutes. We had our first gig at a Beatles tribute show with one of the members of The Choir, and we'd all been stressed about the performance. When he left we opened a bottle of Black Velvet and punched out Pearl Jam's "Porch" for what seemed like forever, guitar solos snaking around rolling snares. Somewhere between the end of that song and the bottom of that bottle, Stacie came back with Kai.

“I don’t understand, or I missed what you said.” I slurred my words. It had been years since I’d had that much to drink.

“It’s dark over there. Six minutes. He asked Lisa, who came to check up on him, how long he’d have if he removed the mask—how long a human can go on with limited oxygen,” Stacie explained. Kai fiddled with the knob on an amp.

“He only has six minutes?” I asked in a drunken panic.

“Not like that,” Eric, one of the guitar players said. “Like hypothetically.”

Six minutes. Just a bit shorter than our version of “Porch,” than a shot or two of whiskey, than my shower the next morning to rinse off the night. Six minutes until the human body will shut itself down. Cease. Forever.

“When?” I asked.

“He’s just asking,” Stacie said. “You know him. He needs to know. He has to know his options. Not tonight. But, he needs to know.”

I nodded, but I didn’t want to stay conscious. I tried to let my eyes roll somewhere else, but they kept returning to the light of the room.

"Do you want an Ativan?" Karen (as she later introduced herself) asked.

"For my dad?" I asked.

"No," she smiled, "for you. It's a sleeping pill. Some people don't want to watch their family members gasping at the end. It will relax you." In disbelief I stared for too long, unable to answer. "It's okay if you don't. I thought I'd just ask." She began to unpack her laptop in the kitchen, and the other bag, most likely filled with the morphine doses needed to sedate my father, was slung around her shoulder. "Shall we?" she asked, gesturing toward the living room.

My dad looked up at Karen when she came in the room and he said with much strength, "You are my comfort."

She smiled and touched his hand, before working her way to the chair on the other side of the room and logging into her laptop. "Your WiFi password?" she asked. None of us could remember. "Never mind, I'll just use my card, but I figured if you had it handy." She went over the doses of morphine we'd already given, logged the information in her computer, and snapped her gum. She explained how she'd begin giving him more doses until the plan was complete.

"Six minutes?" my dad asked.

She nodded.

Mom burst into tears and we all gathered around my dad, to touch some part of his body while it was still warm.

"We'll begin," Karen said. She removed the liquid morphine from the bottle with a syringe, and placed it on my dad's tongue. He received it like communion, the blood of Christ, and closed his eyes, breathing slowly and rhythmically. Aside from the sound of Karen's gum and her fingernails on the keyboard, the room was silent.

We'd begun.

57. More Saints

"What do you think of his plan?" Mom asked me the next day. I knocked on their back door early in the morning. I was awake early; my body was incapable of being "hung over."

We said nothing, but both of us sat in the living room chairs and sobbed. We cried like we did in the beginning, like we'd just found out again. He'd be gone. Soon.

Pa told us to stop. His teeth were chattering—he was always cold, no matter how many blankets we piled on top of him. With no muscle, his body constantly quaked for warmth. He actually smiled, more than he had in months. "Let me die with dignity," he said. "Otherwise it will be a lung infection or something." He breathed. "More pain. Just let me have this one thing while I can still control it." He smiled again.

"Maybe we can make a game out of it for Christmas," Mom said. She laughed, trying to dry her tears. "We can take bets on how long it will take." We bet on everything in our family from Super Bowl to the length of my cousin's relationships.

"Not that long," Pa said. "Soon. Let me do it soon."

Hospice was called and Mom asked if I'd come over for the first meeting to make sure she didn't miss anything. She was a kind-looking young woman, with long brown hair and a gentle face. When she smiled, her eyes lit up. She didn't say much at first, but only asked questions. Pa told her about his mom and how she used to make him eat octopus. He told her how Mom accidentally kicks his legs at night, but he thought it was on purpose. Mom told him to be careful or she'd kick him harder. They laughed. They told stories of the slides and Kai and Stacie and me.

"I can tell you this," the nurse began. "You're not ready."

My dad looked sad. "But I want to die."

"But you're not ready quite yet," she said. "There's too much laughter in this room. You'll know when you can't laugh anymore that it's time. And your body will tell you. I've been in this a while, and every time, the body will let you know."

My dad nodded his head, looking disappointed, but he seemed to trust her. "But when that time comes," he said, "we can do it. Six minutes." She nodded. "Good. That's all I need to know. We can."

"And hospice pays for everything. We will pay for the morphine and the nurse and anything else you need. You just tell us and we'll get it for you. I'm going to leave some morphine with Kathy just in case you need it, but you don't have to pay a dime."

"It's funny," Pa started, then caught his breath. "That the *good* health care only comes at the end."

She smiled, and kneeled next to him, squeezing his hand lightly. "You're lucky to have them." She nodded to us. "And they are lucky to have you. So until your body cries 'uncle,' enjoy these moments."

The room was calm. No one was crying, probably because we felt like she knew us. She understood the dynamic even though she'd only been there a few moments. I'd heard hospice nurses were saints, and she was. Mom had to fill out some paperwork to submit to hospice's care—the hospitals were no longer involved, and all Pa's health care in these finals days was now under the hospice umbrella. There was something both final and calming to it all.

The next few weeks rode on the momentum of the nurse's spirit. We laughed and spent all our time with my dad. It wasn't until I was adding more minutes to Pa's prepaid phone that I realized he may not use them all—that his unused words and time would just sit out there on a phone plan—words left unsaid. So we filled all our time with whatever words we had left. Pa explained over and over how to care for the lawnmower and remove the battery. He was passing on anything he could think of before his body let him know.

The following day I picked up the phone to call Mom, but our line was dead. I shimmied under our deck and found the wires had corroded and separated from the connection. I went to the hardware store for the necessary parts and actually fixed the line—one of the first home improvement projects I'd completed entirely on my own, without any input from my dad.

"You will be okay," Stacie said, comforting me at lunch when I told her about the project. "You will pick up where he left off."

"But I don't want to," I said.

"But you have to."

Later that night Mom called, her voice charged with adrenaline. "Come. Now."

Pa had been having a hard time breathing. He was gasping when I made it over.

"It's not the machine," she said. "It was pushing out air fine. He's just losing it."

He shook his head and gasped quickly. His entire skull pulled back when he breathed. Skin rocking on bone.

"Can't move anything," he whispered. "Just a bit of this hand." He tried to look down, but his head wouldn't respond. Gasps. Mom insisted on transferring him to the bed without me. She said too many bodies made it harder. In bed he still gasped. "Not enough," he said in a broken, hushed voice. "Not enough air." He was panicking.

Mom climbed into bed next to him and stroked his hair. He stared at the ceiling, his eyes filled with terror.

"Go home," Mom said. "I just wanted you here in case something happened. We'll be okay."

When I called the next morning she told me he asked for the morphine—the first time he'd ever, during the duration of the entire disease, asked for any sort of pain medicine. She said his brain was freaking out, convincing him that he was choking, even though he wasn't. But it took a long time for his brain to allow the medicine to work. She finished reading *Travels with Charley* to him. They'd taken to reading every night. That book was one of his favorites—in fact, they were reading the copy he'd bought me when I was in elementary school. "Steinbeck gets it," my dad told me before handing me the book as a kid. I was partial to *Of Mice and Men*, and it was difficult not to think of Lennie's final scene, serenely looking across the river before George pulls the trigger to put him out of his misery.

After they finished the book, Mom pulled up a DVD of their vacation to Nova Scotia on her laptop and the two of them laughed and cried until the morphine took hold, and my dad fell asleep. Mom interrupted herself as she recounted the night. "We never made it to Greenland or Ireland. Those were going to be our next trips. Or Yellowstone at Christmas."

Mom was able to transfer him into his chair in the morning, but just that one dose of the drug knocked him out for the majority of the following day. She tried to rouse him for lunch, but he wouldn't wake up. He finally came to that evening, but struggled. His breathing was off and his eyes were wild. Mom offered him another dose, but he declined it. He was just making sure the morphine would do what he needed it to do. He'd never relied on any sort of medicine. He never asked for a Band-Aid or an Advil. After his hernia surgery he said he'd just "suffer through it. I don't like those drugs."

That night Stacie confessed, "I'm not ready. I'm not. I thought I would be, but I'm not. He's been my dad for all these years. He took me in when no one else would. He loved me like a dad. I can't lose him. I'm never going to be ready for that kind of loss. This is permanent."

Later that evening when I called I asked Mom how long we had until he asked for the mask to be removed. "I don't know. He's suffering. His body is suffering. I can't get him to eat. He can't go to the bathroom. I don't know. Not long."

We received the call the next morning at 4:30 AM that he wanted the mask removed.

"Are you scared?" Karen asked.

It was late now and there was a general calm to the room. We didn't have to say "I love you" anymore because we'd said it all. Every word we'd ever wanted to say to each other had been said. The silence was okay. But Karen's somewhat shrill voice broke that.

I looked at her and frowned. This wasn't the question to ask a dying man.

"No," Pa said rather calmly. I don't think he found Karen as abrasive and uncaring as we saw her. He was so tired of living, that anyone who could help usher him to permanent sleep was a saint. "I'm not scared. I'm actually happy." He quickly said, "No offense to you guys," turning his eyes to us. He smiled. "But I'm happy."

"I'd be scared," Karen said. "I mean, who knows what's on the other side." She snapped her gum. "Good for you, though."

Karen's phone rang. She answered it in the living room. We only heard one side of the conversation. "Hey Kira…No, I have a, thing here…I'm really not sure, but after, yeah I'd love to…I don't know." She leaned forward in her chair to look at my dad, as if she was assessing his death progression. His eyes were closed. "I'm not sure how long."

Mom whispered whatthefuck and said aloud, "You know you can go in the other room."

Karen held her hand to the mouthpiece and said to Mom, "No, I'm fine, thanks." She finished her conversation rather loudly and then hung up, typing more into her computer.

Stacie asked my dad, "Do you want music or us to read to you or anything?"

"No, Sweetie," he replied, "just peace."

Pa looked content in those moments—his eyes closed gently, not in a tight, forced way. The room went quiet, except for the air of the BiPAP, but his breath was slow and regulated. We all leaned, wondering if he was gone. But then suddenly he popped one eye open to look at us, and grinned. He started laughing like the man of my youth—a deep, strong laugh. His adrenaline surely was at work, but it was so good to hear that sound. "You didn't think I lost my sense of humor, did you?" he said.

"I almost forgot," I said, leaping from my spot near my dad. I came back with a few sheets of paper—they were the proofs from my first book. My publisher was kind enough to rush me the pages because he knew my dad was not doing well and I wanted him to see the dedication. I held out the paper in front of Pa. "To Pa, I tried not to use too many adjectives."

He pursed his lips. "It's perfect, kiddo," he whispered. He'd been able to read the whole book in the previous months. And this was the final piece I wanted him to see. "Keep writing. It's important," he said.

"I just wanted you to know." He nodded.

Karen stood up and gave Pa another dose of morphine, the liquid placed on his tongue—this was his seventh (they told us after three doses, he should be out cold, but my dad, even in his final throes, was too strong for seven doses of morphine). Karen dialed out on her phone and began loudly talking about the evening's plans and where she was meeting people.

"My grandson is sleeping—could you go outside or something if you're going to talk like that?" Mom said.

Karen nodded and said to Mom, "That's fine—I'm starving, so I'll see if there is anything in the car."

Before Karen could leave the room, Mom stormed out and went to her bedroom. I could hear her crying. Stacie remained at Pa's feet, so I followed Mom.

"This is all wrong," Mom said. "It's not how it's supposed to be. And she's awful."

"But it's what Pa wants," I said. "And he doesn't know about her—he just wants some peace."

"It's just all wrong."

I went into the kitchen, passing the living room, Pa smiling and talking to Stacie. I heard the words "love" and "daughter."

Karen was ferociously opening a bag of Combos. "Wow, this is my lucky day—I found these in the car. I was so hungry. Sometimes you win, you know?"

Ignoring her every word I said, "So what's Plan B?" She cocked her head. "Because this clearly isn't working—he should be asleep by now, right?"

"I've never seen a patient take so much morphine without some sort of reaction. It's like he's some sort of superhero."

"He is," I replied.

Karen chewed on the inside of her mouth and opened the cellophane wrapper, popping in a Combo. "Do you want to try and remove the mask anyhow?" she asked.

"With him awake?" I said too loudly.

"Well, we could try, see what happens."

I stared into her skull. I breathed so I could compose myself, trying not to scream and wake up Kai. Through gritted teeth I said, "Just so I'm clear, you just suggested we suffocate my father while he's fully conscious. He'd suffer greatly, struggling before us. That's what you just goddamn suggested?" I could feel my eyes growing wild. Karen stopped chewing her Combo.

"Something else. We'll maybe try something else. You're right. There's a stronger sedative, a drip, but I clearly don't have that with me now, but we could try again tomorrow. Because I can't possibly give him any more morphine without an overdose, and then we'd be killing him and we can't do that."

I stared.

"What if he passes out for some reason in the night?" I asked. I realized that Karen couldn't do what my dad needed her to do and I was now faced with the burden of being the one to remove his mask. "Is that legal? Or is that homicide?"

"What are you asking?"

"Can I remove his mask tonight, after you leave, if the morphine were to work? Is that legal or will I go to jail for killing my father?"

"You can. It's legal. We all have documentation of his intentions."

The room was hushed.

"So, are you sending me home?"

I knew I should consult the rest of the family, but I didn't need to—Mom crying in her bedroom, Stacie at Pa's feet—I was doing what they all would want.

"Yes."

Karen immediately pulled out her cell phone and checked the time. Her eyes lightened. She would be able to make whatever social plans she'd been working on in the living room all evening.

"Let me tell him," I said. "Stay here, or pack up, or whatever, but let me tell him." Her bags were already in the kitchen, so she began to shut down her laptop.

I told Mom first. She smiled. "We get him at least another day?" she asked. I nodded. She hugged me. "I want him another day."

In the living room, Stacie hugged Pa's leg. "Hey," I whispered. Pa looked up, his eyes clear. "It's not going to happen tonight." He closed his eyes.

"But it has to," he said. "Sonofabitch."

"The morphine isn't working. You're too strong for it. That body of yours won't shut down, not even now. You're a god."

Pa smiled. "So when?"

"We'll try again tomorrow," I said. "We have some ideas, but you're stuck with us another night." I smiled. So did he.

"They fucked it up, eh?"

"Never trust anyone, right?" That's what he'd always told me about life—never trust someone else to do something right. Just do it yourself.

He grinned.

Aside from Pa, everyone in the room looked relieved. The nightmare hadn't come true. He was alive.

"Will you try to take the mask off while I'm asleep?" he asked me.

"I don't think it works that way, Pops. I think you will wake up."

"I know," he said. "I know." Despite his frail structure, I was relieved to see his chest moving to the beat of the BiPAP. "I can't eat." I didn't care. We'd spend the night and wake up and have him another day.

"You're a badass," Stacie said. "Not even morphine could take you down."

"So..." a perky voice chimed in from the direction of the living room. I'd forgotten Karen was still here. "It was really nice to meet you," she said to Pa. He nodded. It was late—nearing 11:00 PM and he was full of morphine that wasn't working. His eyes looked tired. "And I'm really sorry things didn't work out."

"We're not," I quickly retorted. She understood, I think.

I took the liberty of showing her out of the house, anything to mute her words.

When I came back in Mom had already transferred Pa into bed. "The best one in a while," she said. He wanted to just sleep in the chair, but she insisted he sleep in bed with her.

Stacie and I decided to spend the night—she and Kai on the fold-out bed and me on the couch in the living room. When I went into their room to kiss Pa goodnight he said, before Mom attached the full-face mask, which was easier for him at night, "Sonofabitch, what kind of outfit is this?" He laughed. Stacie and I kissed his head and told him how much we loved him and how happy we were to have another night together.

He smiled and said, "I love you all. So much."

And with that Stacie went to bed with Kai in the next room. I kissed them both and worked my way to the living room, shut off all the lights and covered up on the couch.

I felt like the luckiest man in the world. I could hear Mom giggling in their bedroom. Laughter. Death was scheduled, but it couldn't happen. He was in bed with Mom. He'd be there tomorrow. As grim as the notion was, he'd be there tomorrow. I thought I'd check on him in the middle of the night, just to make sure the morphine hadn't had some sort of delay—just to make sure I shouldn't try to remove the mask. But I knew I wouldn't. I wanted him here. Tomorrow.

Still alive.

Still alive.

58. Sounds

It sounded like a bell. A chime, like the kind small stores hang by their door to alert them a customer has arrived. I jolted awake. I figured the sound was the furnace (though no heat was blowing from the vents) or some other creak houses make; it had been years since I'd slept in my childhood home. The living room was pitch black, but having spent the first twenty-some years of my life in this house, I could navigate it without fail. I pulled the blanket away and sat up. I checked the time on my phone. 3:33 AM. I needed to use the bathroom and figured I'd stick my head into my parents' room to ensure everything was okay. I felt compelled to at least entertain the notion of removing his mask, but I knew if the morphine hadn't worked before, he would still be very conscious.

When I came out of the bathroom, Stacie was standing in the hallway. "Did you hear that?" she asked.

"The bell?"

"No, it was like a quick gasp." I shook my head. "Not a bell, but it woke me up. I wanted to tell you, it's all going to be okay. Last night, when I walked by their room, I poked my head in and your mom was holding his hand, curled up next to him. It was beautiful." I raised my hand because I thought I heard Kai stir. "Did you check on your dad?"

"I'm about to."

She said she'd meet me in there in a minute after she got a drink of water.

There was a soft light coming from underneath my parents' door. I knocked gently, but there was no response. I turned the handle and slowly pushed the door open.

The small lamp with the stained-glass shade was on in the corner, lending a gentle hue to the room, unlike the harshness of the overhead fluorescents. Mom was kneeling on the bed, hunched over my dad. The BiPAP was pushing air in and out of my dad's cheeks. The machine seemed quiet—less intrusive than it had in months. Pa was resting peacefully in the bed. His eyes closed.

Mom looked up when I came in the room. She tried to speak, but it was as if the words weren't there. "Is he. . ." I began.

Mom shook her head. "I don't know. I can't find a pulse."

I quickly rushed to Pa's side of the bed and put my hand on his neck. His skin was warm, but as I moved my two fingers over his neck, I could find no pulse.

Mom looked at me wide-eyed and smiled. "He did it."

Stacie was standing at the door now. "He did it on his own," Mom said. Stacie held her hand to her mouth. None of us cried. He lay there beautiful, warm, and he did it. *Never trust someone to do something right.*

"That's awesome," Stacie said.

"I heard a noise," Mom said.

"What?" I interrupted. "What did you hear?"

"I don't know—it was like shutters flapping. But I woke up and I leaned over and he was breathing, or I thought he was breathing, and, oh, just look at him." Mom picked up his hand in hers. "Just look at him. He's okay. He's peaceful. He hasn't had that kind of peace in a year. And he did it. They screwed it up, as he said, so he did it." We all laughed.

"But how? The mask is still on," Stacie said.

"He just...died. On his own. God," Mom said. "He did it the right way. Like everything else in his life, even in death he did it the right way."

Stacie came next to me and stroked his hair, while I touched his hand. "He's still warm," I said. "It must have just happened."

"What was that sound we all heard?" Stacie asked. The room was silent except for the machine.

"Shut it off," Mom said. "Let him be free finally of that thing."

I reached over and clicked off the power. His cheeks were still now. Mom undid the straps of the mask. He was beautiful without the mask. It had been so long since we'd seen him without it—only during a transfer. Always briefly. But there he lay. Beautiful. I kissed his head.

"I'm so happy for him," Mom said. "He did it his way. No drugs left in his system. No nurses. There was no gasping. God, I didn't want him to go that way last night. But this...well, this...it's absolutely perfect."

The tears began, but not out of sorrow or loss; those would stream in the upcoming hours, days, months and years. But those tears at that moment that swelled and rolled down our cheeks were tears of joy for my dad who did it right, like everything in his life. He did it right.

59. Now What?

"Now what?" I asked. We'd been laughing and telling stories about my dad. His skin grew cold as we gathered around him. Mom said she knew what killed him—she said as she changed for bed that night she flashed him and his eyes grew wide and he smiled. We laughed.

"I should call hospice. And you should go pick up Grandma and bring her over here."

When she made the call, it wasn't anything like the practice runs—the panic and repetition. There was a lightness in her voice.

"Is it okay that I'm happy for him?" I asked Stacie.

"Of course. He'd want it like this. He was a superhero. Even in death."

Stacie went back into bed to be with Kai, and I left Mom to have her time with her husband. The roads were abandoned. It was the day before Thanksgiving, 4:30 AM. Many people had that day off and were sleeping in. The car's radio played Pearl Jam's "Yellow Ledbetter": *And I know, and I know, I don't wanna stay.*

Grandma held a handkerchief to her eyes the entire drive.

"Was it peaceful?" she asked.

"It was perfectly peaceful," I said. "In his sleep. He went in his sleep."

When we arrived, Grandma went into the bedroom, kneeled by the bed and began to pray. I gave her the privacy she needed. Hospice was there quickly. The nurse was an angel—every stereotype of the kindness that this organization exudes was embodied in her words and movements. She was the antithesis of the previous night's experience.

After speaking in a soothing hush, she pulled out a stethoscope and explained she had to verify this passing. "My dad would want that," I said. "He told me to make sure he was dead." She laughed. Grandma cried in the living room, the only light from three candles on the piano, while the three of us tended to Pa. The room was quiet as the nurse listened to Pa's chest.

"So peaceful," the nurse said, touching Pa's hand. "No signs of any distress whatsoever. We could all wish for our last moments to be like his."

"Was it an overdose of the medicine?" I asked. "Or something else?"

"I looked at the logs this morning," the nurse explained. "All of those drugs were out of his system before he even went to bed, and they were actually low doses. This was all him. He died on his own."

The nurse explained that the funeral home would come to pick up my dad. She never used the word "body." He was always a person, even in death. She then worked methodically in the kitchen to crush the many bottles of leftover medicine and mix the liquid morphine into a bag mixed with flour. "I'll miss him," I said to her. I don't know why, but I felt like I could tell her. "I already miss him." The happiness of his peaceful passing was slipping into true mourning—the kind that sticks in your throat and lungs and won't dislodge. I joined Grandma in the dark living room. She didn't say anything. Typically, I would console or at least speak. But I didn't want to. I was comfortable in the silence of the flickering candles.

When she was done with the pills, the nurse told Mom that she would go in to clean my dad before the funeral home arrived.

"Let me," Mom said. "I want to."

"It's one of the last, most loving acts someone can do. Most people don't want to, but I am always touched and can tell how close a couple is when this happens."

Mom cleaned Pa and changed his clothes. She was crying when she came out. Stacie embraced her.

White reverse lights filled the living room as the funeral van backed into the driveway. Two men introduced themselves, offered their condolences, and then wheeled a gurney into the bedroom. They calmly explained everything. They offered us our last time with Pa. Grandma went in and then Stacie. Mom said she was content. "We will now go in to place Daniel on this gurney and take him to our vehicle. We are required by state law to wear gloves when we do this. I just want to let you know, because it's upsetting to some people." Mom said she understood.

As the men wheeled the cart down the hallway, I interrupted, "Can I help?"

They both turned and the man who originally spoke said, "Of course."

I couldn't imagine Pa leaving the house with these two men in latex gloves. I wanted to touch his skin, like he would know. They were kind, explaining how to lift his body and make the turn onto the gurney. "1, 2, 3," said the man. We lifted, but exerted no energy because Pa was so light now. His body was already stiff and cold and far gone from that moment when we all first found him. As we walked down the hall, I kept a hand on my dad, but once we reached the door, I knew I'd have to let go. The men lifted the cart and Mom propped open the door. The coldness rushed inside, and for the first time in over a year, Pa left the house. And we cried. We sobbed and we hugged and we cried. The house felt wrong, like it lacked windows or a foundation or walls. It felt foreign and strange—almost clinical. Pa's decline was messy, filled with machines and transfer boards. This new place felt bleached and abandoned. The light was too bright.

Mom put together some kind of breakfast, after which Grandma asked to be taken home. And we cried.

It wasn't until I returned that Kai awoke. "Papa?" he asked, touching the seat where my dad had been for nearly Kai's entire life. "Where is Papa?" Kai asked.

I didn't know how to explain it. My throat was locked with grief. So Mom said, "The moon. Papa is on the moon now, watching us."

Kai looked at her, back at the seat, then returned to her. "Okay," he said.

I wanted that kind of contentment.

We filled the next few hours with business—calling those that needed to know, leaving messages with insurance agents. As the day ticked by the four of us sat in the living room unable to function. "This isn't good," Stacie said, after we had been sitting in silence for nearly twenty minutes. "I have no idea what to do or how to function." We nodded. "Call Debbie," Stacie said. "She'll know what to do." Debbie had been Mom's closest friend. She and Mom met when Jenny, her daughter, and I were in school together. They'd been through it all together. Debbie was just like my dad—practical and sensible.

Mom smiled, "You're right."

Debbie was over in what seemed like seconds. She hugged us, but didn't gush. She wasn't there to cry, but to offer advice. "It's like Dan is back," Stacie said.

Our biggest issue was simply what to do. "I'll go with you to the funeral home," Debbie said. She had been making pies for the next day, but put them on hold to help us out and make decisions when we began to emotionally shut down.

When we were done and returned home Debbie said, "Now, we need to figure out Thanksgiving." We'd been offered many homes and meals when we called people, but none of it felt right. My aunt had to leave the previous night to see her kids in California. Mom told her to go, that there was nothing else to be done. But we lacked a place to be for the meal the next day.

"I can't imagine making all that food and just sitting in this house," Mom said.

"Then don't," Debbie said. "Make some of it—whatever is easy and go somewhere else new. Like the lake park Dan loved so much. Go there."

"But what if it rains?" I asked. They had been predicting storms.

"Then sit in your car. Just go somewhere that feels right."

She was right. So, Stacie, Kai and I went home to prepare cranberries. The next morning, I put together the corn custard and Tofurky (our traditional vegetarian replacement). Mom worked on the mashed potatoes and stuffing. She brought over tinfoil cake pans and we made servings for each person—all mashed into one tin. We laughed and remained focused. We had to. When we stopped, we ceased functioning. So we moved.

By the time we picked up Mom, the sun had begun to set and it was gray and cloudy. When we reached the lake park it was storming huge raindrops, so I transformed my car (the Honda Element was able to recline all the seats into a giant bed). The four of us sat crossed-legged in my car with our plates of food and had a Thanksgiving meal.

"Oh, what they will think of our family when Kai goes to preschool and tells everyone that his family had Thanksgiving in the car."

I turned on the stereo and played "Alice's Restaurant" through my iPhone. It was a tradition in our family to listen to this eighteen-and-a half-minute-long song every Thanksgiving. Pa could recite the entire thing by memory. "The twenty-seven eight-by-ten color glossy pictures with the circles and arrows and a paragraph on the back of each one explaining what each one was." He'd crack himself up every time he said the lines.

"I think Pa timed it so he could get out of Thanksgiving," I said.

Mom and Stacie laughed. "I had the same thought when I was making the stuffing," Mom said. "He hated Thanksgiving. He said the food all sucked and he'd rather eat pierogies."

"He hated all holidays," I said.

"I loved and hated that about him," Mom said. "He'd get so angry when people came over, but his reasoning was so sweet, too. He'd say, 'I just like it when they're gone because then I can have the people I really love, you and Mike and Stacie and Kai, all to myself.' He was always that way. Even when Mike was a kid, he hated this day."

"Can I tell you something, though," Stacie said. "Is it wrong that this feels like the best Thanksgiving I've ever had—I mean, besides the obvious? Just being here with only you guys?"

"Of course you think that," Mom said. "You're Dan junior. That's why he always loved you the most."

"That's not true," Stacie protested.

"Oh come on, Stacie," I said. The moment he met you, we all became second, third and fourth in his lineup. He adored you like his own."

Stacie started crying. "I miss him."

"But you're right," Mom said. "I was teasing you, but this feels right."

Kai asked for more Tofurky, and I took some from my tin and placed it on his. The windows were fogged up from the heat of the meals. The parking lot where we sat was abandoned; everyone else was with their families. Suddenly headlights flashed into the car. I wiped the steam from the windows. "Is it the cops?" Mom asked. "Because if we get arrested, that is going to make for a bad day."

"Worse than it already is?" I asked. She smiled.

It wasn't the cops, only a car turning around.

The rain let up for a few moments, so we threw all of our containers into the garbage cans and walked around the now-dark lake park. "He loved it here," Mom said. "This is right." We all held onto one another tightly, like if we held on enough we wouldn't feel the void, the missing presence. But we did. We would for the rest of our lives feel that hollowness.

"No moon," Kai cried, pointing to the sky. It was cloudy and began to rain lightly again. "So no Papa?" he asked.

"Nah, buddy, he's here," I said. "I feel like he's here tonight."

60. The Details

The business of death is business, but we navigated it the best way we knew. Mom told the funeral home not to order an urn. Brian, her friend Penny's husband, was a custom wood worker, so he constructed a beautiful box from curly maple to hold Pa's ashes. "This is the most important gift you could have given us," Mom explained to him. He was humble and said it was nothing. But it was something extraordinary. His work was fine and the details were exquisite. "This is where Dan would want to be," Mom said.

We skipped the church and the funeral home all together. Instead we had a celebration—a party at the local nature and science center that housed huge conference rooms, but also snakes and fish and honey bees on the other side of the building. "Dan would want this," Stacie said. "He'd want Kai to be entertained and to be connected with the animals. This is who he was." We had the celebration fully catered with French food to celebrate his heritage—cheeses and breads and pastries and endless bottles of wine. We filled the tables with pictures and played music I pulled from his computer, a night for Pa. On the night of the party Cleveland was pounded with a ferocious snowstorm, but that did not dissuade a single person that mattered from coming. The room was packed—Diane, the woman who cut his hair, dozens upon dozens of people Pa worked with, one of my old college professors whom Pa befriended, Mom's friends, and on and on and on. People laughed and ate. They cried when David gave a speech about my dad and their friendship. They cried when I played the video I'd made of my dad, a series of pictures of him put to the soundtrack of Eddie Vedder's "Man of the Hour."

After the party died down, a few of us gathered the few undrunk bottles of wine. There was no food left because people celebrated as they should have. The night, despite the hardship of missing my dad so greatly, was the closest any of us felt to him since he'd died. He felt alive and real and tangible again. "Can you imagine," Mom said on the way home, "if we'd had this in a church or funeral home? It would have been awful. This was something special." And it wasn't just extraordinary for us, because Mom received thank you cards for months after the party from people thanking her for "doing it right." They said seeing that much love in one room was an important moment in their lives. David wrote me, "Mike - Just wanted to say, again, that your dad would be proud and grateful for the way you helped us all send him off with a smile and some laughter. Thank you for that. And know that if you ever feel like you want to talk the energy out of any of this, I'm available. And you need to come visit that old guitar sometime. Peace – David."

Another guest wrote my mom, "I told my husband that when I die I want that—that exactly. I want a celebration, not a funeral."

It was exactly what we all needed to feel close.

But it wasn't enough.

When the people were gone and there was no longer a party to plan or pictures to organize it was easy to lose my dad. Stacie and I no longer discussed the afterlife as we had extensively when he was still alive. I knew she didn't believe, and I wasn't that far off, though I still had a shred of hope that there was something more—not pearly gates or any religious rhetoric, but I hoped we went back into the cosmos or energy field or whatever. I'd always hung onto Einstein's theory I learned in physics in high school, "Energy cannot be created or destroyed." Stardust. Something. I hoped that still applied, but I was losing my faith because without evidence, I was without my dad.

I thought a lot about Saint Thérèse—wondering if that moment in that church could ever happen—if I would ever see my dad again in the wind of the oak tree or twisted in the rays of the streetlight outside our house. I tried to find him when I'd walk through the backyard at night from Mom's house—in the darkness I said, "Now you could come and I won't be afraid." I felt a slight shiver as I passed over the walkway I built and past the shed doors my dad and I constructed together. But he never came.

One afternoon, shortly after his death, the lyrics to a Train song I never really listened to (one of those white noise songs that's on in department stores and waiting rooms) came into my head: "I need a sign to let me know you're here / All of these lines are being crossed over the atmosphere." I was standing on my deck looking out at our backyards, angry. He should have come back by now. Saint Thérèse was a hallucination. Death was final. Ashes to ashes. Dust to dust. I was desperate for a sign—man is weak like that. The stories of Jesus' miracles, though most likely a fabrication of man, were created because without them, faith is too much of a task. We rely on the tangible. *I need a sign to let me know you're here.*

I don't know why I darted inside. I don't know why I walked past Kai, who was asking for me to play with him, or didn't respond to Stacie when she asked where I was going with such determination. But I went into her office, opened up her display case that housed the bowl we bought on our honeymoon and other souvenirs. At the bottom was a small frame with an image of a palm and a child resting on the hand. It also displayed the scripture: "See! I will not forget you…I have carved you on the palm of my hand. Isaiah 49:15." My dad had given it to Stacie when I first met her. She and my dad would talk about everything: politics, personal matters, and religion. By all intents and purposes he was the father she'd never really had, and he gave her this gift in a small frame once, saying he'd always be there for her. She cried when he gave it to her.

I tore it apart. The frame had dust on the top, resting without notice in this case for years. I flipped it over and pulled up the metal prongs that secured the piece of cardboard and the image in place. I flicked the cardboard insert on the ground. Words. Behind the image was a small slip of paper filled with words for Stacie. I wiped my eyes on my sleeve. "Stacie," I cried. "Stacie!"

She looked panicked when I stumbled into the living room. "What's wrong?" she asked.

"This," I said. "Have you ever looked behind that palm picture in your room from Pa?"

"What do you mean look behind it?"

"Did you ever tear it apart?"

"I don't understand. Why would I tear it apart? That's the frame he gave me."

"I know. Did he ever say anything about a note to you? In the picture?"

She shook her head.

"Look, I said. "Read. For us—for you. He's okay, I think."

Stacie,

Life isn't always easy, so many decisions to make, so many paths to follow. As you go through life believe in God and pray to Him every day. He will always answer your prayers. He will guide you through events and people, listen and watch for Him, He is there.

Love Ya,

Pops Hemery

She finished reading and looked up at me. "I think he did it. I think your dad came back to tell us he was okay. I don't believe in anything else, but..." She hesitated. "But I believe in your dad."

61. Final Visits

I didn't hear from him again until Kai was in the hospital being treated for severe dehydration. He had come down with a particularly awful strain of the flu and couldn't keep down fluids. After trying to insert an IV into his arms and feet eleven times, they eventually put a tube in his nose and down his throat to get some liquid back into his body. It was awful—worse than watching my own father die. Stacie and I were emotionally ruined. We were sitting in the hospital room when my cell phone rang. It was sitting on the counter across the room—when I picked it up the caller ID said "Dan Hemery" with a picture of him. We'd long ago deactivated his phone and his number was sold off to someone new. But there it was—plain as could be.

"Hello," I said. Silence. "Hello? Are you there?"

There was no one on the other end, but I refused to hang up until it disconnected. "Can you hear me?"

"Who is it?" Stacie asked.

"My dad?" I showed her the phone log, recent calls: Dan Hemery. She smiled.

"The man is good. He knows when we need him," she said.

Epilogue

Kai is nearly six years old and we now have a new addition to the family, Vivienne, our highly-active three-year-old daughter. She never met my dad, but she holds his name within hers: Vivienne Kathleen Daniella Hemery. We thought it would be a nice way to keep Mom and Pa together longer.

Mom is strong; she tends to her yard work with the dedication of my father, though no one can weed a backyard like he did. She keeps the house tidy, just as my dad did—hollering at us when we leave cups on the table or toys in the living room. Her basement walls are filled with pictures of her and my dad, vacations to the east coast and a trip to the Cheers bar in Boston. Vivienne knows the person in the pictures is Papa, even though she's never had the joy her brother experienced of sitting on his lap shouting, "Car."

We talk about him all the time. His presence is there in stories and pictures. "I miss him," Kai says sometimes.

"Good." I always respond the same way. I make him tell me the stories of sitting on his Papa's lap over and over so they imprint into his permanent narrative. Even if it's just the story and not the actual memory, that's fine.

Pa doesn't show up much anymore. For a while I thought maybe he was speaking through my stereo. I realize there are institutions for people who believe the dead are speaking through their stereos—but it seemed like songs would be timed out perfectly. Our anthem for the illness, Pearl Jam's "Just Breathe" always seemed to come on when we needed it. I wonder if sometimes these appearances are me simply looking too deeply, trying to find him in self-made metaphors. Or maybe he's always there, but I only notice when I'm looking for him.

The last time he showed up was at a Barnes & Noble. The kids were looking for books and Stacie and I were fighting about money. She bought an expensive coffee from Starbucks and a quilting magazine, and we were short on cash (granted, my frugality is legendary). I was angrily saying that this wasn't the month to splurge while she said we both made enough money to buy a coffee. We were cutting each other down in the children's section of the book store when suddenly I heard someone speaking French with the same thick accent my dad had—something authentic. We both stopped arguing and turned to see a dark-haired, late-thirties man with a square face sitting on a step reading to his beautiful blond daughter in French. The language, which I will forever regret not learning, was reminiscent of my youth, my dad and my grandparents at parties with the other relatives. The scene was too beautiful, this man and his daughter, the language shared between them. She responded in French, her voice small and cute, as she cuddled into his arms.

"Your dad," Stacie mouthed to me.

He read to her for a long while. Kai and Vivienne read next to us, but we just sat there, listening to this man's voice. Stacie squeezed my hand. "Kind of reminds you what matters, huh?" she said.

I nodded and squeezed her hand.

Stacie packed up the kids, helped them with their jackets and went with them downstairs to pay for the books they picked out. "I'll be right there," I said.

The man was kneeling next to the little girl, helping her with her jacket.

"Pardon," I said. The man looked up and smiled. "Parlez-vous anglais?"

"Yes," he said.

"I'm so sorry, but I overheard you speaking French to your daughter, and it reminded me of my dad. And I wanted to thank you."

"My wife," he began, "is French. She wanted our kids to be bilingual so we try as much as possible."

"Thank you," I said. "Your accent was spot on, like my dad. Thanks for letting us hear him again tonight."

The man smiled, his eyes light and caring like my father's.

***

Kai and I lie beneath the same tree in my mom's front yard where I used to lie with my dad. Kai is neatly tucked into my arm as I was with my father. This is where my dad and I watched my kite fly all day and into the evening when it got stuck on the wires across the street. Pa said it was even better because we didn't have to even hold the kite, but could watch it sail. Kai and I just finished playing baseball—he's good, really good, a genetic gift from his mother. The shade is cool, offering the same respite it did when I was a child.

"What do you see?" I ask Kai. My dad used to ask me the same question. The clouds dance above us, shape shifting at will.

"That one," Kai says, pointing, "a boat!" He's excited because he's right. It's a boat—but only for a moment before it changes into something else. "Oh," he says with disappointment. "It's gone now."

"But it's something else," I say. "Everything is always changing—sand castles get swept away in the tide and flowers open and close throughout the day. Just because they change doesn't mean we don't enjoy them. So what is the cloud now?"

"A French fry?"

I laugh because he's funny. He has a keen sense of humor that honestly makes me laugh whenever he speaks. "And that's cool, too, right?"

"Not as cool as a boat." He's right about that, too. Change happens all the time, and it's not always as cool. My dad's absence in our lives isn't a positive change. At all. I try to keep him alive through stories—the ones before he was sick. But the stories mixed with illness are the only ones Kai can remember, so I let him share those when he wants to talk about my dad.

Mom is having a rough time some days. There is that initial relief of not having to be a caregiver full time and being able to get the mail and not wonder if he'll be alive when she returns. But after that wore off she was only left with ghosts and memories that slip and shift like the clouds. We visit often, probably too often. I walk the same steps my dad walked, mimic his fathering, the way my kids tuck into my arms. My dad's life has always been entwined with mine. When he was alive we twisted and grew around one another—he taught me how to be a man, and I think I pushed him to reevaluate parts of his life, like being a vegetarian and questioning organized religion.

I hate myself when I fail to live in his shadow, when it takes me six hours instead of one to fix the broken pipe on the back of our house. But I also have come to terms with being my own man. I'll never be able to build Kai a darkroom, like my dad did for me, the drywall perfect and the plumbing complicated. But in the end, there isn't much I can do. My dad was right—we all will end up at the same place—the only difference is how we get there.

Therefore, I plan on getting there the best way I can, with my two kids nuzzled under my arms and my wife by my side. Because no matter how much planning, worrying (and I worry greatly about life's trials) and calculating, it can all fall apart just like that.

So we go.

"A pineapple!" Kai yells. "No, no, a tower with syrup and a donkey running next to it." He speaks quickly—I can feel his body vibrating next to mine as he tries to keep up with the clouds. "It's all too fast," he moans. He speaks like an adult. "A monkey, no a hill with a car and a piece of candy. I can't possibly keep up."

"You don't need to," I say. "We'll miss some of the stuff, but just relax and shout out the coolest things you see, each and every one."

Acknowledgments

I can't tell this story without thanking the following people. Without them, I would have emerged at the other end of this thing with many more permanent scars and lost the will to turn on the computer every morning to hammer out the words about those days: Lisa and the kind folks at the ALS Association, hospice, Kathy Hemery (I'm glad you're swearing less these days), Stacie Leatherman for being with me for every breath and allowing me to learn from your infinite patience and wisdom, Kai, Vivienne, Jack Hertvik (the first one I told about the disease—by saying it aloud, I could begin to understand it), almost everyone in chapter 6 (I was angry, I'm sure you understand), Eric Anderson (let's get the band back together—that's easier than writing), Ryan Vana for every letter you stuffed in my mailbox to try and make this thing right, all of my students who have read my books (and those who now understand satire by mocking my author photo obsessively), Sean Folk for introducing my book to so many of the United States national parks (and FedEx drivers), Sue William Silverman for telling me to keep going when all I wanted to do was quit, Bob Babcock/David Ingle/all the folks at Deeds Publishing for believing in this project with such enthusiasm, and all the souls who have or will walk these steps in some form. Find peace. It is there, tucked in those moments.

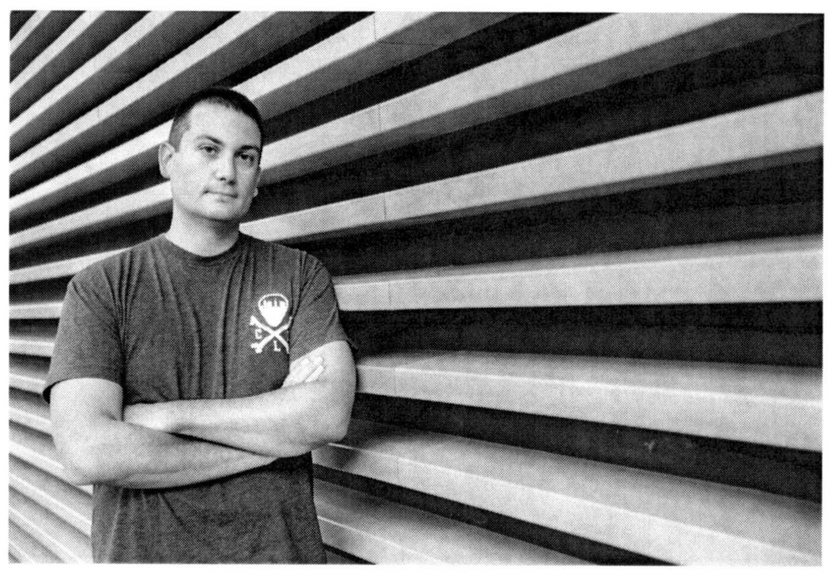

MICHAEL HEMERY is the author of one previous book, *No Permanent Scars*, a nonfiction short-story collection. He has also been published in *Drunken Boat*, *Los Angeles Review*, *Lumina*, *New Plains Review*, *Passages North*, *The Portland Review*, *Post Road Magazine*, *Redivider*, *Slice*, *sub-TERRAIN*, *The Tusculum Review*, and the book *Fearless Confessions: A Writer's Guide to Memoir*.

Hemery, who earned his MFA from the Vermont College of Fine Arts, is a high school English teacher. He also served as the nonfiction editor for *Hunger Mountain*. He resides in the Cleveland area with his family.